Augmentative and Alternative Communication Intervention

An Intensive, Immersive,
Socially Based Service Delivery Model

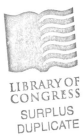

Augmentative and Alternative Communication Intervention

An Intensive, Immersive,
Socially Based Service Delivery Model

Janet L. Dodd
SLP-D, CCC-SLP

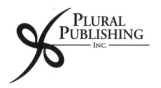

PLURAL
PUBLISHING
INC.

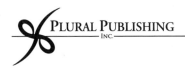

5521 Ruffin Road
San Diego, CA 92123

e-mail: info@pluralpublishing.com
Website: http://www.pluralpublishing.com

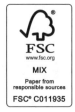

FSC
www.fsc.org
MIX
Paper from
responsible sources
FSC® C011935

Typeset in 11/13 Palatino by Flanagan's Publishing Services, Inc.
Printed in the United States of America by McNaughton & Gunn, Inc.

Library of Congress Cataloging-in-Publication Data

Names: Dodd, Janet L., author.
Title: Augmentative and alternative communication intervention : an intensive, immersive, socially based service delivery model / Janet L. Dodd.
Description: San Diego, CA 92123 : Plural Publishing, [2018] | Includes bibliographical references.
Identifiers: LCCN 2017017272 | ISBN 9781597567251 (alk. paper) | ISBN 1597567256 (alk. paper)
Subjects: | MESH: Communication Aids for Disabled | Communication Disorders--rehabilitation | Communication | Interpersonal Relations
Classification: LCC RC428.8 | NLM WL 340.2 | DDC 616.85/503--dc23
LC record available at https://lccn.loc.gov/2017017272

Contents

Preface

The intervention approach described in this book merges the author's experiences working as a school-based speech-language pathologist (SLP) and training aspiring graduate student clinicians. Through her experience as a school-based SLP, she recognized the inadequacies of current models in meeting the intervention needs of many of the students on her caseload. In spite of employing what was deemed best practices in working with students with complex communication needs (CCNs), many of these students remained bereft of communication.

Initially devised as a means to provide communication sciences and disorders graduate student clinicians with hands-on experience, Chapman University's *All About Communication* (*AAC*) Camp evolved into an exemplary alternative school-based service delivery model. Striving to emulate a camp experience, *AAC* Camp is provided to students with CCNs as a component of their extended school year (ESY) program. ESY refers to special education and related services (e.g., speech-language intervention, occupational therapy) that are provided to a student beyond their normal school year in order to prevent the excessive loss of skills or deterioration of behavior that is likely to occur in the presence of an extended break (Individuals with Disabilities Act [IDEA], 2004). In participating schools, select students, referred to as campers, leave their special education classes to attend "camp" for two weeks where they participate in various camp-themed activities, including daily camp fire time, nature hikes, scavenger hunts, and arts and crafts. Graduate student clinicians who assume the roles of "communication guides" scaffold communication opportunities within these experiences while employing language stimulation techniques. These techniques include modeling, expansionism, and self-talk through the application of aided language stimulation and augmented input to create a language-rich immersive environment. Utilizing a child-centered approach (Paul & Norbury, 2012), communication guides teach campers to use core vocabulary across a wide range of activities, expanding the purposes for which they communicate (Dodd & Gorey, 2013; Dodd & Hagge, 2014). Campers' response to the intervention is monitored throughout the two-week period. Given this intense block of intervention, students with CCNs are able to firmly establish newly acquired skills. The purpose of this book is to introduce this alternative, school-based service delivery model that was devised to address the unique needs of students with CCNs.

The intervention model discussed in this book is designed to facilitate a novice AAC user's communication skills by guiding them in acquiring skills and strategies in using their AAC systems effectively, while progressing them towards increased levels of communicative competence (ASHA, 2004; Light, 1989; Light & McNaughton, 2014). This is accomplished by utilizing natural interactions and experiences and immersing the child in his or her AAC language. The intervention model described in this book enhances successful communication and minimizes social barriers (e.g., language gap) by providing training and support to communication partners and guides.

CHAPTER 1: INTRODUCTION

There is a subgroup of children within the category of individuals with CCNs for whom developing even the most fundamental aspects of communication is an arduous task. These children are the focus of the intervention model described in this book. This chapter describes the intervention needs of these children and explains why current intervention approaches (e.g., PECS, Milieu Training, Functional Communication Training) are failing to meet their needs. This chapter also highlights the importance of essential aspects of communication as discussed by key researchers in the field of AAC and autism (Light, 1989; Wetherby & Prizant, 1989). Common AAC myths will be dispelled once and for all.

CHAPTER 2: INTERVENTION AS A PROCESS

Intervention, particularly as it relates to AAC, is a dynamic process—constantly shifting in response to a student's reaction to the intervention and their changing communication needs. This dynamic process is best conceptualized by Schlosser, Koul and Costello's (2007) adaptation of Garlund and Björck-Åkesson's (2005) definition of intervention as a "a super-ordinate concept for the different intentional steps taken to change the behaviors or attitudes of person interactions, procedures, events or environments in a desired direction" (p. 232). Intervention, as it reflects this definition and pertains to AAC, is a series of intentional steps taken towards an identified goal. In this case, the goal is to establish a language-rich environment to support the novice AAC user's achievement towards greater levels of communicative competence. These intentional steps, referred to as phases, are based on, and include, activities related to assessment, intervention planning, and ultimately implementation of the intervention (Schlosser, Koul, & Costello). This chapter will introduce the intensive, immersive, socially based intervention model, which is the focus of this book, including a brief description of each phase of the intervention process.

CHAPTER 3: ASSESSMENT PHASE

The purpose of assessment is threefold: (1) determine if a student would benefit from an AAC system; if so, (2) identify the appropriate AAC system based on the student's abilities and communication needs, and (3) guide educational planning. This chapter will provide specific details regarding the assessment phase of the intervention process, including a discussion regarding how AAC assessments differ from traditional assessments of speech and language skills. An overview of different assessment models and their contribution to the intervention process is included. The final section of this chapter will discuss how to apply information gleaned from assessment to the intervention planning and implementation phases.

CHAPTER 4: INTERVENTION PLANNING PHASE

This chapter focuses on the planning phase of the intervention process. The chapter begins with a discussion of the different types of vocabulary, and the rationale and importance of teaching core vocabulary, while gradually expanding a student's fringe vocabulary. Symbol sets and systems are discussed, as well as how consistent placement of icons assists students who have difficulty with picture discrimination. Strategies to create a symbolically rich environment so the student with CCNs can be immersed in his/her language system throughout their day are reviewed. Included are strategies to adapt children's stories to make them more meaningful to symbolic communicators. The importance of training support staff on key components of this intervention model and a training outline are shared.

CHAPTER 5: INTERVENTION IMPLEMENTATION PHASE

The overarching goal of AAC interventions is to improve AAC skills (Binger, Berens, Kent-Walsh, & Taylor, 2008). An AAC-based intervention approach not only promotes AAC skills, but facilitates acquisition of communication skills, supports a student's understanding of language, and improves oral language. This chapter presents the intervention implementation phase, including application of language-based intervention strategies to AAC. Example lesson plans are provided and instructional strategies are outlined.

CHAPTER 6: PROGRESS MONITORING

Progress monitoring, as it relates to students with disabilities, is the scientific practice of assessing a student's progress and evaluating the effectiveness of an intervention (IDEA, 2004). Monitoring a student's progress is not only good clinical practice, but a mandate under federal law (IDEA, 2004). This chapter will discuss the importance of progress monitoring as it relates to the intervention process, including how to write goals across Light's (1989) four competency areas. This chapter includes sample goals and progress-monitoring strategies, complete with suggestions for collecting and reporting students' progress.

CHAPTER 7: CASE EXAMPLES

The longest of the seven chapters illustrates the intervention approach from theory to practice. The case examples presented in this chapter will illustrate the implementation of the intervention program described in this book with nine students. The students in these case examples represent children with a range of diagnoses and disorders, each with their own unique set of communication needs. Key aspects of the intervention process are highlighted throughout each case example.

HOW TO GET THE MOST FROM THIS BOOK

Whether you are interested in running an AAC Camp or Clinic for your students, or just want to learn how to more effectively work with students who are learning to communicate through the assistance of AAC, this is the book for you! It is strongly suggested you read through the entire book to really understand all the components that go into planning and implementing an evidence-based AAC intervention. Then continue to use this book as a resource as you develop a similar program for your students. Examples of how to develop present levels of performance (PLOPs) are presented throughout Chapter 3 and embedded in the case examples shared in Chapter 7. Additionally, use the goals presented throughout these two chapters to develop individualized educational plans (IEPs) for your students. In the appendices you will find examples of how to develop your own adapted stories and activities that really work with this population. Also included in the appendices are resources you will refer back to again and again. On the accompanying PluralPlus companion website, you will be able to download forms you can use for the purposes of data collection and progress monitoring, as well as a sample letter you can send home to parents to inform them how to use the "School-to-Home" book, bridging what you are doing with their child at school, to home.

REFERENCES

American Speech-Language Hearing Association [ASHA] (2004). *Roles and responsibilities of speech-language pathologists with respect to augmentative and alternative communication. Technical report.* Retrieved from http://www.asha.org/policy/TR2004-00262/

Dodd, J. L., & Gorey, M. (2014). AAC intervention as an immersion model. *Communication Disorders Quarterly, 35*(2), 103–107. http://dx.doi.org/10.1177/1525740113504242

Dodd, J. L., & Hagge, D. (2014). AAC camp as an alternative school based service delivery model: A retrospective survey. *Communication Disorders Quarterly, 35*(3), 123–132. http://dx.doi.org/10.1177/1525740113512670

Individuals with Disabilities Education Act, 20 U.S.C. § 1400. (2004).

Light, J. (1989). Toward a definition of communicative competence for individuals using augmentative and alternative communication systems. *Augmentative and Alternative Communication, 5*(2), 137–144.

Light, J., & McNaughton, D. (2014). Communicative competence for individuals who require augmentative and alternative communication: A new definition for a new era of communication? *Augmentative and Alternative Communication, 30*(1), 1–18.

Paul, R., & Norbury, C. F. (2012). *Language disorders from infancy through adolescence: Listening, speaking, reading, writing, and communicating* (4th ed.). St. Louis, MO: Elsevier Mosby.

Schlosser, R. W., Koul, R., & Costello, J. (2007). Asking well-built questions for evidence-based practice in augmentative and alternative communication. *Journal of Communication Disorders, 40*, 225–238.

Acknowledgments

Thank you to all the children with complex communication needs (CCNs) who challenged me to do things better.

Thank you to my graduate students whose creativity helped me expand my ideas and for taking what you learned to change how services are provided to children with CCNs in public school settings.

Thank you to Judy Montgomery, my colleague, mentor, and friend. You always encouraged me to think outside of the box and inspired me to convert my ideas into actions.

Most of all, thank you to my husband and my children, Chase and Ryder. You were always there to support and encourage me.

CHAPTER 1

Introduction

Communication is the essence of human life.
—Light, 1997, p. 61

Communication is an innate, complex task that most of us don't think much about. It just happens; in fact, we do it all day long with little attention to how we do it or why we do it. This seemingly effortless act is wrought with challenges for those with the most complex communication needs (CCNs). Children (and adults) with a wide range of disabilities face many challenges associated with the quintessential act of communicating. Individuals with CCNs— which is how they are collectively referred to in the field of augmentative and alternative communication (AAC)—find this innate task unsurmountable. So who are these children with CCNs? Children with CCNs are not children with a specific diagnosed disorder, but rather a cluster of children whose disabilities significantly impair their ability to access communication via traditional means (i.e., oral language). It is not a single disability but a variety of disabilities with one thing in common: an absence of functional communication. Children with CCNs may have a diagnosis of autism, Down syndrome, cerebral palsy, or intellectual impairment. Each child's individual challenges hinder their ability to develop functional communication skills (Dodd & Gorey, 2014).

There is a subgroup of children within this broader category for whom even developing the most basic communication skills, such as those necessary to fulfill immediate wants and needs, is an arduous task. Children with the most severe forms of autism are often among these individuals. Children unable to develop a functional form of communication often present with severe deficits in receptive and expressive language skills and poorly measured levels of cognition, which are further compounded by deficits in social communicative functioning (SCF) (Dodd, 2010). Examples of SCF in an emergent communicator include the ability to establish joint attention, respond to bids for interaction, and initiate interactions (Dodd, 2010; Dodd, Franke, Grzesik, & Stoskopf, 2014). These, often undeveloped, skills severely impact the ability of students with CCNs to use their communication systems. Nonetheless, in spite of intense efforts to apply what has been deemed evidence-based practice (EBP) in working with children with CCNs, both in theory and practice, there remains a cluster of children bereft of communication skills.

The single most important skills we can teach an individual with CCNs is communication. Exceeding the ability to write one's name, sort objects by color, and imitate motor gestures, communication is directly associated with greater levels of independence. These children not only need to gain access to a means to communicate, they have to learn how to communicate, and more importantly, they need to develop a sense of the value of communication. The intervention model described in this book blends what we know about evidence-based practices related to working with children who are learning to communicate with the support of AAC, and those with autism and other developmental disabilities.

AUGMENTATIVE AND ALTERNATIVE COMMUNICATION

Many children with CCNs will inevitably rely on augmentative and/or alternative forms of communication at some point in their lives, either to support their development of oral language, supplement their oral language, or as their primary means of communication. The International Society for Augmentative and Alternative Communication (ISAAC, 2016) describes AAC as:

> a set of tools and strategies that an individual uses to solve everyday communicative challenges. Communication can take many forms such as speech, a shared glance, text, gestures, facial expressions, touch, sign language, symbols, pictures, speech-generating devices, and so forth. Everyone uses multiple forms of communication based upon the context and our communication partner. Effective communication occurs when the intent and meaning of one individual is understood by another person. The form is less important than the successful understanding of the message. (https://www.isaac-online.org/english/what-is-aac/)

Communication boards, electronic speech-generating devices (SGDs), gestures, and sign language are all examples of AAC. The American Speech-Language-Hearing Association (ASHA, n.d.) describes AAC as:

> . . . all forms of communication (other than oral speech) that are used to express thoughts, needs, wants, and ideas. We all use AAC when we make facial expressions or gestures, use symbols or pictures, or write. People with severe speech or language problems rely on AAC to supplement existing speech or replace speech that is not functional. Special augmentative aids, such as picture and symbol communication boards and electronic devices, are available to help people express themselves. This may increase social interaction, school perfor-

mance, and feelings of self-worth. AAC users should not stop using speech if they are able to do so. The AAC aids and devices are used to enhance their communication.

As these definitions demonstrate, AAC can take many forms based on the needs of the individuals. For the purposes of this book, the term "communication system" will be used as a generic term in reference to any type of communication system, including non-technology-based communications systems such as communication boards and books, along with high-tech dynamic display type communication systems. For a review of terms related to AAC refer to Table 1–1.

Use of Terms to Describe Early Communicators

A number of terms have been used to describe students (and adults) who are in the early stages of developing communication skills. Early communicators (one such term) use both symbolic and non-symbolic forms of communication, with or without communicative intent (Beukelman & Mirenda, 2013: Snell, 2002; Wetherby & Prizant, 1989). Wetherby and Prizant, based on their research, concluded that communicative behavior, including both symbolic and non-symbolic forms of communication, is considered intentional "if the individual has an awareness or mental representation of the desired goal" (p. 77). Maladaptive behaviors such as hitting, biting, or throwing oneself on the floor serve various communicative functions, such as to escape or avoid an unpreferred activity. They are frequently non-intentional on the part of the communicator. Communicative acts such as these become "communicative" in nature based on adult elucidation of communicative intent (Wetheryby & Prizant, 1989). That is, adults impose meaning to these behaviors (e.g., "Oh he doesn't want to come to the table") and respond accordingly. Repeatedly responding to non-intentional, non-symbolic behaviors in a consistent manner reinforces the continued use of these behaviors for obtaining a desired outcome to the point that these non-symbolic forms of communication become intentional on the part of the communicator. Examples of non-symbolic forms of communication include eye gaze, gestures, vocalizations, facial expressions, body language, and behaviors. Manual signs, picture symbols, and words are examples of symbolic forms of communication (Beukelman & Mirenda; Snell; Wetherby & Prizant). Given this dichotomy of terms, the following terms are proposed to describe the abilities of early communicators: *pre-intentional non-symbolic communicator*, *intentional non-symbolic communicator*, and *intentional symbolic communicator*. Intervention teams may find using these terms helpful in explicitly describing the communication skills of early communicators.

In addition to *early communicator*, the terms *beginning communicator*, *emergent communicator*, and *emergent AAC communicator* are often applied to

Table 1–1. AAC Terms

Term	Definition
Unaided Communication Systems	Gestures, body language, and sign language are examples of unaided communication systems. Unaided communication systems rely on the user's body as a means to convey messages.
Aided Communication Systems	Aided communication systems encompass both technology- and non-technology-based tools and strategies that a communicator uses to aid with communication.
Dedicated System	A dedicated system refers to equipment specifically designed to operate as a communication aid.
Speech-Generating Device	A speech-generating device (SGD), also referred to as a voice output communication aid (VOCA), is an <u>electronic augmentative and alternative communication (AAC)</u> system with voice output capabilities. These types of communication devices allow the user to select words or messages to be spoken out loud. There are a wide variety of SGDs available, ranging in complexity and cost.
Digitized Speech Output	A time-sampled replication of actual human speech. Live recordings the AAC user can use in the context of a communicative interaction. Generally speaking, digitized speech is more natural sounding than synthesized speech in terms of pitch, resonance, and prosody.
Synthesized Speech Output	Letters, words, or symbols that are translated into computer-generated speech. Most high-tech SGDs offer a range of computer-generated voices to allow the AAC user to choose their voice.
Traditional Grid Display	Traditional grid displays organize symbols in columns and rows, frequently by parts of speech. This type of display can be used to promote sentence structure and word order.
Cell	This is an area on a device that corresponds to a vocabulary item or message, and can be selected and activated. The term "button" is sometimes used synonymously. For the purposes of this book, the term "cell" will be used.
Selection Technique	This is a method an AAC user uses to identify or select items on their communication systems for the purposes of communication. The two primary selection techniques are direct selection and scanning.
Direct Select	This is a selection technique in which the AAC user directly selects or activates an item on their communication system through pointing. The AAC users who use direct selection frequently use their index finger, a pointer, or eye-tracking technologies to select desired icons.

continues

Table 1–1. *continued*

Scanning	Scanning is a selection technique frequently used by individuals with significant motoric limitations, who are unable to independently directly select items. In this technique, items in the selection set are highlighted or scanned. When the desired icon is reached, the AAC user indicates their desire for the highlighted item through the most easily accessible method, such as head nodding, vocalization, or activation of a switch.
Static Display	Static or fixed display communication systems are low-tech communication systems in which the location of symbols remain constant. The total number of cells an AAC user has access to is limited to the number of symbols that can fit on a single page. Given an opportunity to engage in a different topic or activity, the AAC user would need to switch to another page. This generally requires the assistance of a facilitator. GoTalk and 7-Level Communicators are examples of low-tech fixed display communication systems.
Dynamic Display	Dynamic display communication systems are high-tech communication systems in which individual cells, when activated, can link to other pages. These were once considered only an option for cognitively competent AAC users, however, with early exposure to advanced technologies such as the iPad, this technology is very intuitive to young AAC users.

Source: Definitions adapted from Beukelman & Mirenda, 2013.

those who are acquiring communication through the use of AAC. According to Beukelman and Mirenda (2013), *beginning communicators* refers to individuals who use non-symbolic forms of communication, either intentionally or non-intentionally, to fulfill immediate wants and needs. Also, within this categorization are individuals who are emerging in their use of symbolic communication (i.e., aided or unaided forms) to convey basic messages, as well as individuals who are emerging in their use of AAC technologies. Additionally, they use the term *emergent AAC communicator* to describe individuals who present with profound delays in the areas of language and cognition secondary to severe neurological trauma. Frequently, all modalities of language and cognition are affected. These individuals require intervention approaches to assist them in understanding and gaining control of their personal environment. These particular individuals need to begin by developing foundational, or precursor skills, prior to the introduction of AAC. Review of available resources indicates the terms *beginning* and *emergent communicators* are often used synonymously to describe individuals, children, and adults, who are developing the skills necessary to establish themselves as communicators.

The author of this book would like to suggest the use of a term to recognize children who are "verbal" but not yet communicative: *functionally nonverbal*. Students who have learned scripts and readily imitate (echolalic) are often described as being verbal when in application or functionality they are not. Labeling a child such as this as "verbal" can, in fact, hinder their progression towards becoming a spontaneous verbal communicator. It is not uncommon for others to assume because they are "verbal" they are communicative and therefore not a candidate for AAC. However, given the visual support of an AAC system such as a low-tech communication board or book, many of these children can and do learn how to use oral language functionally. Refer to Myth #3 for further discussion regarding the fallacy of this direction of thinking.

For the purposes of this book, the terms *beginning* and *emergent communicator* are used to refer to students in general who are in the early stages of developing their communication skills. If a more specific or descriptive term is warranted, then one of the other terms will be used.

WHAT ARE THE INTERVENTION NEEDS OF STUDENTS WITH COMPLEX COMMUNICATION NEEDS?

Students with complex communication needs, particularly those who are the target of the intervention presented in this book, need an intervention program that capitalizes on their strengths, and advances them toward greater levels of communicative competence. Communicatively competent individuals use communication effectively to manage their environment and engage in meaningful interactions. Students with autism and other communicatively hindering disabilities possess strengths in their ability to make sense of information conveyed in a visual medium (Mesibov, Shea, & Schopler, 2005). In fact, many of these students gravitate and demonstrate improved performance when information and expectations are expressed to them visually in forums such as visual schedules and choice boards. In addition to maximizing visual supports, students with CCNs who are in the emergent stages of learning to communicate need an intervention that:

◆ Embraces a developmental approach to language acquisition
◆ Builds vocabulary skills recognizing the significance of early acquired words
◆ Extends communication skills beyond requesting preferred food items and objects
◆ Fosters independent use of their communication system
◆ Uses visual supports to model language and create a language-rich environment
◆ Blends evidence-based practices for working with children learning to use AAC and children with autism and other developmental disabilities
◆ Teaches application of communication within naturalistic contexts

CURRENT TREATMENT APPROACHES

Students with complex communication needs are exposed to a myriad of treatment approaches with varying degrees of success throughout their educational careers. As many of these students matriculate through school, it is not uncommon to witness a recycling of interventions that were previously attempted. Picture Exchange Communication Systems (PECS), Functional Communication Training (FCT), and Milieu Training are among the most commonly used teaching approaches used with students with autism and other communicatively impairing disabilities.

Picture Exchange Communication System (PECS)

The Picture Exchange Communication System (PECS) is a naturalistic approach to teach children with autism and other developmental disabilities how to communicate. PECS, introduced by Bondy and Frost in 1994, encourages children to spontaneously initiate communication within a social context using primarily direct reinforcement. It was developed to assist children with significant communication deficits in acquiring functional communication skills. Children learn to spontaneously initiate their desires by exchanging corresponding picture icons for desired items. "Children learn to approach a communicative partner in order to request a desired item. Once this skill is learned, PECS use is expanded so that children develop a broad vocabulary, sentence structure, and additional communicative functions" (p. 742). Successful implementation of PECS is dependent on the correct identification of a child's preferred reinforcer (Ganz, Simpson, & Lund, 2012).

Unlike other communication approaches, students who have difficulty with imitation skills, facial orientation, or motor skills can learn PECS (Bondy & Frost, 1994). It can be easily implemented with few materials at a reasonable cost (Ganz et al., 2012). Picture icons are created based on the student's preferences. The ease of implementation and portability of this approach makes it a preferred communication option. Students develop functional communication skills and are able to request what they want and need by exchanging picture icons in response to adult questions or prompts (Sulzer-Azaroff, Hoffman, Horton, Bondy, & Frost, 2009).

Functional Communication Training

Children who are unable to communicate will find ways to fulfill their immediate wants and needs. Unfortunately, students who have limited communication skills frequently employ maladaptive behaviors (e.g., screaming, hitting themselves, biting, and breaking objects) as a form of communication, particularly when their needs are met in response to those behaviors (Casey & Merical, 2006). Functional communication training (FCT), developed in the

1980s, teaches students more appropriate means to communicate their needs and wants (Carr & Durand, 1985). FCT begins with a functional behavior assessment (FBA) to identify inappropriate behaviors and the functions of those behaviors. Applying the principle of functional equivalence (Beukelman & Mirenda, 2013; Durand, 1990) the student is then taught more acceptable replacement behaviors that serve the same function (Mancil & Boman, 2010). The key to successful implementation is replacement of aberrant behaviors with more acceptable behaviors that are equally successful in achieving the desired outcome.

FCT, as described by Kurtz, Boelter, Jarmolowics, Chin, and Hagopian (2011), is "a well-established treatment" to reshape inappropriate behaviors that are used to "maintain attention, access to tangible items, and escape from demands" (p. 2940) into more socially acceptable behaviors. For example, if a child is getting snacks when he hits himself to calm him, then he will continue to engage in hitting when he wants to eat. If his hitting behavior does not allow him to obtain snacks, he will eventually stop hitting. Additionally, instead of acknowledging his hitting behavior, FCT teaches him to use an acceptable form of communication, such as saying or signing, "Eat." By increasing the student's communication skills, there should be a noted decrease in the occurrence of maladaptive behaviors (Mancil, Conroy, Nakao, & Alter, 2006).

Milieu Teaching

Milieu Teaching (MT) is defined by Kaiser (1993), as "a naturalistic, conversation-based teaching procedure in which the child's interest in the environment is used as a basis for eliciting elaborated child communicative responses" (p. 77). Milieu Teaching is a naturalistic approach that teaches communication skills to children with autism and other communication-impairing disorders. In this approach, children are provided with support to facilitate generalization of learned behaviors across different settings and people (Warren & Gazdag, 1990). Learning of communicative behaviors occurs in naturalistic settings, optimizing incidental teaching opportunities that are supported through the use of mand-modeling and delayed prompting or time delay. (Christensen-Sandfort & Whinnery, 2011). In MT, children learn effective ways to request preferred objects or activities within the context of naturalistic interactions (Goldstein, 2002).

Given a naturally occurring communication opportunity (i.e., incidental teaching), the adult uses a series of graduated prompts (e.g., 30-second delay, prompt to request—either gesturally or verbally, direct imitation), always starting with the least restrictive, to facilitate the elicitation of the target behavior. If the child fails to demonstrate the target behavior given a communication opportunity paired with a time delay, the adult either models the target behavior or mands (requests) the behavior (Yoder et al., 1995). While these procedures facilitate acquisition of requesting behavior, the incidental teaching procedure paired with the time delay is dependent on the child initiating the communicative act. Comparatively, mand-modeling is reliant on the adult controlling the learning.

Children increase their frequency of communication and generalize newly learned skills across people and settings (Yoder et al., 1995). MT is directed by a child's interests; therefore, adults must be able to recognize a child's interests in order to capitalize on teachable moments. In studies, MT is a practical and cost-effective communication intervention that teachers can embed into class activities for children with autism and other communication-impairing disorders (Christensen-Sandfort & Whinnery, 2011).

WHY DO CURRENT TREATMENT APPROACHES FAIL?

The primary goal of AAC-based interventions for students with severe disabilities is to improve functional communication skills, enabling them to participate in a wide range of activities and environments with an expanding range of communication partners (Calculator, 1999). As Light (1997) suggests, functional communication includes the ability to express wants and needs, establish social closeness, exchange information, and participate in routines of social etiquette. The abovementioned behavior-based interventions help children with CCNs develop functional communication skills to satisfy their needs and wants, transitioning them from pre-intentional, non-symbolic communicators to intentional symbolic communicators. However, through this vertical progression of communication—pre-intentional to intentional and non-symbolic to symbolic—many of these interventions fail to advance these individuals on the horizontal dimension of communication (Wetherby & Prizant, 1989). For example, an emergent communicator who progresses from using the manual sign for "more" to using four symbols to construct the sentence, "I want red skittles" demonstrates growth on the vertical dimension of communication but not on the horizontal dimension of communication. There is a failure to expand communication skills at the horizontal level, which may be typified by increasing their vocabulary set, introducing novel sentence constructions, or extending their pragmatic use beyond requesting.

The overarching goal of these behavior-based interventions is to improve the student's ability to communicate for functional purposes, and in some cases, decrease aberrant behaviors. For example, PECS is often utilized to increase children's requesting capabilities. Children develop a form of communication by exchanging picture icons of desired items and/or actions to gain access to those items and/or actions, which is dependent on the child having the particular picture icon needed for the communicative exchange (Flippin, Reszka, & Watson, 2010). FCT focuses on teaching children to replace maladaptive behaviors with more appropriate and socially acceptable forms of communication. However, several studies found that although there was a reduction in the use of maladaptive behaviors, very few of the participants actually increased their symbolic communication skills, including spoken words (Mancil, 2006). Although MT supports children's generalization of learned skills in naturalistic environments, there remain limitations with regard to expanding their communication skills. Students may develop the ability to communicate their desires across different people and settings; however, they remain deficient in social skills and spans of communication skills. The most critical limitation of these interventions is lack of opportunities to cultivate the horizontal dimension of communication, which will support students with CCNs in developing communication skills that extend beyond fulfilling immediate wants and needs.

COMMUNICATIVE COMPETENCE

The goal and philosophical foundation of the intervention described in this book is to facilitate the emergence of competent communicators. Communicative competence is grounded in the development and integration of knowledge, judgment, and skills in four interrelated domains: linguistic, operational, social, and strategic (Light, 1989). Competent communicators portray a positive self-image and show interest in their communication partners (Light, 1997). In order to accomplish this, they initiate interactions, actively participate, and take turns in a symmetrical fashion (Light, 1997). Competent communicators demonstrate responsiveness to their communication partners and become participants in the communication process by making relevant comments, asking partner-focused questions, and negotiating shared topics (Light, 1997). Just as typical communicators express their wants, needs, desires, thoughts, arguments through verbal communication, AAC users do the same through the use of their communication system. The intervention approach described in this book helps students who use AAC to become competent communicators using their communication system so they too can participate in the quintessential act of communication.

Communicative competence enables the AAC user to regulate the behavior of those within their immediate environment by communicating their wants and needs. But that is not all! A competent communicator is one who (a) shares information about personal (e.g., what they did over the weekend) or upcoming events (e.g., a pending trip to Disneyland); (b) greets classmates in the morning; (c) acknowledges accomplishments of others; (d) conforms to routines of society; (e) expresses preferences; and (f) engages in all aspects of the communicative process including initiating and terminating conversations and introducing conversational topics of personal interest (Beukelman & Mirenda, 2013; Light, 1997). In order to support students with CCNs to achieve greater levels of communicative competence, it is imperative for beginning communicators to develop AAC skills in each of the four competency areas identified by Light (1989) in her definition of communicative competence: linguistic, operational, social, and strategic competencies.

◆ Linguistic competence refers to the receptive and expressive language skills of one's native language(s), as well as knowledge of the linguistic code unique to their AAC system (e.g., line drawings and words).
◆ Operational competence refers to the technical skills needed to operate the AAC system accurately and efficiently.
◆ Social competence includes the skills of social interactions such as initiating, maintaining, developing, and terminating communication interactions.
◆ Strategic competence involves the strategies used by people who rely on AAC to compensate for the functional limitations associated with the use of an AAC device (Light, 1989, Light & McNaughton, 2014).

It is imperative that as a part of the intervention process, skills are targeted in each one of these competency domains. We never know the level to which a beginning communicator will achieve communicative competence until we get there, but without setting high expectations we will never know how far they can go.

MYTHS BUSTED!

One of the barriers hindering students' access to appropriate and effective interventions are misconceptions. A misconception or false belief is an incorrect assumption that is reached, in part, because of a lack of understanding or misinformation. As misconceptions are repeated, they gain momentum to the point of being accepted as fact. Over the years several myths have transpired regarding AAC and individuals with CCNs. The following discussion will, hopefully, alleviate some of these misconceptions and assist in substantiating the truth through a review of relevant research, ultimately resulting in better access for individuals who could benefit from AAC-based interventions.

Myth #1: AAC Will Inhibit the Development of Speech

When the option of AAC is first suggested to a parent of a child struggling to develop oral language, it is not uncommon for them to respond with mixed emotions. Parents can be reluctant to embrace the concept of an AAC system for their child simply out of fear it will impede their child's ability to ever develop speech. Worse yet, to them, is a feeling that we (the intervention team) have given up hope that their child will ever develop speech, even though that is generally not the case. There is a misconception that if a child is exposed to an alternative form of communication, such as a communication book consisting of pictures, we have in some manner abandoned the pursuit of oral language. The opposite is actually the truth; alternative forms of communication actually supporting the development of oral language (Harris & Reichle, 2004; Romski & Sevcik, 1996).

Research shows that AAC does not inhibit the acquisition of speech (Millar, Light, & Schlosser, 2006; Schlosser & Wendt, 2008). In fact, there is evidence to suggest AAC may support the acquisition of speech and language in some children. A meta-analysis conducted by Millar et al. (2006) examining the effects of AAC on the speech production skills of individuals with developmental disabilities concluded that none of the individuals in the studies reviewed demonstrated decreases in speech production. Whereas 11% showed no changes in speech production skills, 89% of the participants demonstrated gains in speech. Further debunking this myth is a systematic review conducted by Schlosser and Wendt (2008) in which they examined the effects of AAC on the speech sound production skills of children with autism spectrum disorder (i.e., autism and pervasive developmental disorder—not otherwise specified). Once again, AAC-based interventions did not impede the acquisition in speech. In fact, many of the studies examined reporting increases in speech production in response to the AAC interventions in many of their participants.

It has been postulated, based on current research, that AAC use may support the acquisition of speech, in part due to expanding the AAC user's ability to participate in conversational interactions, while simultaneously reducing the physical demand or pressure to speak (Blischak, Lombardino, & Dyson, 2003). Speech-generating devices (SGDs) possess additional benefits of providing immediate output. As Romski and Sevcik (1996) suggested, the acoustically consistent production of words provided by a SGD promotes improved attention and, ultimately, imitation of verbal models delivered from the AAC system. Likewise, the pairing of graphic symbols with synthetic speech provides the AAC user with additional opportunities to hear messages within the presence of their graphic counterpart, strengthening the emergent communicator's grasp of the relationship between graphic symbol and spoken word association (Blischak et al., 2003).

The last aspect related to the fallacy that AAC will inhibit speech production applies to the principle of efficiency (Beukelman & Mirenda, 2013). This principle states that individuals will "communicate in the most efficient and effective manner available to them at any given point" (p. 226). If the AAC user is capable of using speech, they are going to use speech. Students with CCNs will use the quickest and most effective means available to them to communicate.

Review of the relevant data supports the notion that in some individuals, AAC may actually facilitate acquisition of oral language by giving users more opportunities to interact with peers and those within their immediate environment, thus increasing their language skills, and providing a frequent and consistent model for speech. Therefore, it is the responsibility of intervention teams to educate parents and families regarding the added value of AAC.

Myth #2: The Child Is "Too Low" To Be Considered for an AAC System

There is a perception that there is a group of children for whom AAC should not be considered as a viable option because they are somehow identified as being "too low" or "too impaired." It is important for us, as professionals, to recall that even very young children engage in purposeful, communicative behavior well before the development of oral language. So why is it that we hold children with CCNs to almost a higher standard before considering alternative means to support their language development? There is a misconception that a student must possess certain prerequisite skills prior to being considered a candidate for AAC. Among these "prerequisite skills" are communicative intent, understanding of cause-effect relationships, and demonstrating interest in others. These are among the very skills that can be taught through AAC-based interventions (Kangas & Lloyd, 1988). Although there appears to be a relationship between cognitive skills (e.g., understanding cause and effect, and means to an end relationship) and language and communication skills, this is not an absolute relationship in which one set of skills precedes the other or vice versa (Kangas & Lloyd, 1988; Romski & Sevik, 1996). However, as Romski and Sevik point out, due to this intertwined relationship between cognition and language, failing to give students access to a means to communicate may further hinder their cognitive development.

Additional prerequisite skills deemed cursory for AAC use (particularly technology-based systems) include the ability to categorize similar objects, match symbols and objects, and exhibit memory for recall. Contrastively, there is emerging evidence to suggest that children with the most complex communication needs can learn to access words and messages not based on categorical understanding (e.g., understanding that playground slides are found in playgrounds) or object-to-symbol identification, but rather by learning and establishing specific motor movement patterns. This is similar to the manner in which we learn to use a computer keyboard by never having to look at the keys as we type. Additionally, we acquire linguistic skills, such as semantics and syntax, by using them (Goossens', 1989). There does not exist any predetermined skills an individual most possess prior to being a candidate for an AAC system. As Cress and Marvin (2003) state, "AAC is applicable at all ages for learning communication roles and behaviors as well as for functional communication for persons who do not yet demonstrate clear referential symbol use" (p. 254).

Myth #3: Only Individuals Who Are Completely Nonverbal Benefit from AAC Systems

There is a common misconception that if an individual "speaks," there is no need for an AAC system. This myth has direct application for both adults with acquired disabilities (e.g., traumatic brain injury, stroke) and children who struggle with expressive language due to motor constraints such as those diagnosed with apraxia of speech or cerebral palsy. These individuals may not have as many of the compounding factors (e.g., impaired cognitive abilities, social communication deficits) as the students who are the focus of this book, but they, too, benefit from AAC support. Many of these individuals with residual speech can communicate more effectively when provided with AAC support.

This myth is also applied to students who present as functionally nonverbal (a term introduced earlier in this chapter). Students with CCNs, who are the focus of this book, may present with "some speech," and are, therefore, overlooked as candidates for AAC because they "speak." Although, as previously discussed in this chapter, individuals who are identified as "functionally nonverbal students," benefit considerably from AAC. AAC helps these students bridge the gap from engaging in verbal behaviors, such as verbal stim (e.g., reciting excerpts from a movie or cartoon) or echolalia, to using oral language for communicative purposes. AAC provides the visual support many of these students need to connect oral language to communication.

Consider the following case study: Nathan, a 6-year-old boy who could imitate anyone and everything, but yet could not initiate use of language for functional means, such as requesting puzzle pieces (one of his preferred activities), craft supplies to complete a craft project, or comment about preferred and nonpreferred activities. Nathan was introduced to a 7 × 7-grid communication board consisting of core vocabulary words. The bottom row of his communication board included colors. There were activity-based fringe strips that could be changed depending on the current activity. Although Nathan could not initiate verbal language, when given the visual support of this AAC system—a communication board and activity specific fringe strips—Nathan quickly learned to use oral language to engage in the various activities presented throughout his day. Nathan progressed from being a functionally nonverbal student who only imitated and recited movie scripts, to being a verbal communicator who shared experiences and participated in activities with peers. Thus, AAC should be considered not only as a means to communicate, but a means to teach communication (Dodd & Gorey, 2014).

Other Myths

There are a number of other myths that serve as barriers to those with CCNs gaining access to the intervention they need. The consideration that AAC should only be considered as a last resort for someone who is unable to develop oral language is unsubstantiated by research. The key to responding to these misconceptions is to understand the intricacies and impact that communication has on the quality of the life of those who possess it. Individuals who use AAC have demonstrated significant gains in behavior, attention, independence, self-confidence, class participation, academic progress, and social interaction. And with regard to AAC hindering one's use of oral language, recall a person who is unable to communicate will find other ways to communicate. Therefore, it is important we teach these individuals appropriate, meaningful, and effective means to communicate.

WHAT TO EXPECT WITH THE REST OF THIS BOOK

Students with CCNs need a goal-driven intervention program that is methodically and systematically planned out, taking into consideration their strengths and weaknesses, and building upon those to achieve a desired outcome—in this case, increased levels of communicative competence. The intervention approach presented in this book bridges evidence-based practices between working with individuals who use AAC to those practices effective in meeting the needs of students with autism and other developmental disabilities. The intensive, immersive, socially-based service delivery model presented in this book links clinical practice to research, providing students with CCNs an intervention model that supports their acquisition of communication skills, not only on a vertical trajectory but on the horizontal dimension of communication as well. As stated by National Joint Committee for the Communication Needs of Persons With Severe Disabilities (1992), the translation of intervention goals to practice, "means teaching communication forms and functions—with the functions discoverable only in the interactive, socialized contexts in which these functions occur and are responded to by other people" (http://www.asha.org/njc). It is for this reason that intervention for students with the most complicated communication needs involve direct therapy within a naturalistic, social context. The intervention approach described in this book aims to do just this, and progress students with CCN toward greater levels of communication competence.

REFERENCES

American Speech-Language-Hearing Association. (n.d). *Augmentative and alternative communication (AAC)*. Available from http://www.asha.org/public/speech/disorders/AAC.htm

American Speech-Language-Hearing Association. (2005). *Roles and responsibilities of speech-language pathologists with respect to augmentative and alternative communication* [Position statement]. Available from http://www.asha.org/policy

Beukelman, D. R., & Mirenda, P. (2013). *Augmentative and alternative communication: Supporting children and adults with complex communication needs* (4th ed.). Baltimore, MD: Paul Brookes.

Blischak, D., Lombardino, L., & Dyson, A. (2003). Use of speech-generating devices in support of natural speech. *Augmentative and Alternative Communication, 19*(1), 29–35.

Bondy, A., & Frost, L. (2001). The Picture Exchange Communication System. *Behavior Modification, 25*(5), 725–744. http://dx.doi.org/10.1177/0145445501255004

Bondy, A. S., & Frost, L. A. (1994). The Picture Exchange Communication System. *Focus on Autism and Other Developmental Disabilities, 9*(3), 1–19. http://dx.doi.org/10.1177/108835769400900301

Calculator, S. N. (1999). AAC outcomes for children and youths with severe disabilities: When seeing is believing. *Augmentative and Alternative Communication, 15*(1), 4–12.

Carr, E. G., & Durand, V. M. (1985). Reducing behavior problems through functional communication training. *Journal of Applied Behavior Analysis, 18*(2), 111–126.

Casey, S. D., & Merical, C. L. (2006). The use of functional communication training without additional treatment procedures in an inclusive school setting. *Behavioral Disorders, 32*(1), 46–54.

Christensen-Sandfort, R. J., & Whinnery, S. B. (2011). Impact of milieu teaching on communication skills of young children with autism spectrum disorder. *Topics in Early Childhood Special Education, 32*(4), 211–222. http://dx.doi.org/10.1177/0271121411404930

Cress, C. J., & Marvin, C. A. (2003). Common questions about AAC services in early intervention. *Augmentative and Alternative Communication, 19*(4), 254–272. http://dx.doi.org/10.1080/07434610310001598242

Dodd, J. L. (2010). Thinking outside of the assessment box: Assessing social communicative functioning in students with ASD. *ASHA Division 16: Perspectives on School Based Issues, 11*(3), 88–98.

Dodd, J. L., Franke, L. K., Grzesik, J. K., & Stoskopf, J. (2014). Comprehensive multidisciplinary assessment protocols for autism spectrum disorder. *Journal of Intellectual Disability: Diagnosis and Treatment, 2,* 68–82.

Dodd, J. L., & Gorey, M. (2014). AAC intervention as an immersion model. *Communication Disorders Quarterly, 35*(2), 103–107. http://dx.doi.org/10.1177/1525740113504242

Durand, V. M. (1990). *Severe behavior problems: A functional communication training approach.* New York, NY: Guilford Press.

Flippin, M., Reszka, S., & Watson, L. R. (2010). Effectiveness of the picture exchange communication system (PECS) on communication and speech for children with autism spectrum disorders: A meta-analysis. *American Journal of Speech-Language Pathology, 19,* 178–195.

Ganz, J. B., Earles-Vollrath, T. L., Heath, A. K., Parker, R. I., Rispoli, M., J., & Duran, J. B. (2012). A meta-analysis of single case research studies on aided augmentative and alternative communication systems with individuals with autism spectrum disorders. *Journal of Autism and Developmental Disorders, 42,* 60–74.

Ganz, J. B., Simpson, R. L., & Lund, E. M. (2012). The Picture Exchange Communication System (PECS): A promising method for improving communication skills of learners with autism spectrum disorders. *Education and Training in Autism and Developmental Disabilities, 47*(2), 176–186.

Goldstein, H. (2002). Communication intervention for children with autism: A review of treatment efficacy. *Journal of Autism and Developmental Disorders, 32*(5), 373–396.

Goossens', C. (1989). Aided communication intervention before assessment: A case study of a child with cerebral palsy. *AAC Augmentative and Alternative Communication, 5,* 14–26.

Harris, M. D., & Reichle, J. (2004). The impact of aided language stimulation on symbol comprehension and production in children with moderate cognitive disabilities. *American Journal of Speech-Language Pathology, 13,* 155–167.

International Society for Augmentative and Alternative Communication. (2016, June 1). *What is AAC?* Retrieved from https://www.isaac-online.org/english/what-is-aac/

Kaiser, A. P. (1993). Parent-implemented language intervention: An environmental perspective. In A. P. Kaiser & D. B. Gray (Eds.), *Enhancing children's communication: Research foundations for intervention* (pp. 63–84). Baltimore, MD: Paul H. Brookes.

Kangas, K., & Lloyd, L. (1988). Early cognitive skills as prerequisites to augmentative and alternative communication use: What are we waiting for? *Augmentative and Alternative Communication, 9*(1), 3–9.

Kurtz, P. F., Boelter, E. W., Jarmolowicz, D. P., Chin, M. D., & Hagopian, L. P. (2011). An analysis of functional communication training as an empirically supported treatment for problem behavior displayed by children with intellectual disabilities. *Research Developmental Disabilities, 32*(6), 2935–2942. http://dx.doi.org/10.1016/j.ridd.2011.05.009

Light, J. (1989). Toward a definition of communicative competence for individuals using augmentative and alternative communication systems. *Augmentative and Alternative Communication, 5*(2), 137–144.

Light, J. (1997). "Communication is the essence of human life": Reflections on communicative competence. *Augmentative and Alternative Communication, 13,* 61–70.

Light, J., & McNaughton, D. (2014). Communicative competence for individuals who require augmentative and alternative communication: A new definition for a new era of communication? *Augmentative and Alternative Communication, 30*(1), 1–18.

Mancil, G. R. (2006). Functional communication training: A review of the literature related to children with autism. *Education and Training in Developmental Disabilities, 41*(3), 213–224.

Mancil, G. R., & Boman, M. (2010). Functional communication training in the classroom: A guide for success. *Preventing School Failure, 54*(4), 238–246.

Mancil, G. R., Conroy, M. A., Nakao, T., & Alter, P. J. (2006). Functional communication training in the natural environment: A pilot investigation with a young child with autism spectrum disorder. *Education and Treatment of Children, 29*(4), 615–633.

Mesibov, G. B., Shea, V., & Schopler, E. (2005). *The TEACCH approach to autism spectrum disorder.* New York, NY: Plenum/Kluwer Academic.

Millar, D. C., Light, J. C., & Schlosser, R. W. (2006). The impact of augmentative and alternative communication intervention on the speech production of individuals with developmental disabilities: A research review. *Journal of Speech, Language, and Hearing Research, 49,* 248–264.

National Joint Committee for the Communication Needs of Persons with Severe Disabilities. (1992). *Guidelines for meeting the communication needs of persons with severe disabilities* [Guidelines]. Available from http://www.asha.org/policy or http://www.asha.org/njc

Romski, M. A., & Sevcik, R. A. (1996). *Breaking the speech barrier: Language development through augmented means.* York, PA: Brookes.

Schlosser, R. W., & Wendt, O. (2008). Effects of augmentative and alternative communication intervention on speech production in children with autism: A systematic review. *American Journal of Speech-Language Pathology, 17,* 212–230.

Snell, M. E. (2002). Using dynamic assessment with learners who communicate nonsymbolically. *Augmentative and Alternative Communication, 18,* 163–176.

Sulzer-Azaroff, B., Hoffman, A. O., Horton, C. B., Bondy, A., & Frost, L. (2009). The Picture Exchange Communication System (PECS): What do the data say? *Focus on Autism and Other Developmental Disabilities, 24*(2), 89–103. http://dx.doi.org/10 .1177/1088357609332743

Warren, S. F., & Gazdag, G. (1990). Facilitating early language development with milieu intervention procedures. *Journal of Early Intervention, 14*(1), 62–86. http:// dx.doi.org/10.1177/105381519001400106

Wetherby, A. M., & Prizant, B. M. (1989). The expression of communicative intent: Assessment guidelines. *Seminars in Speech and Language, 10*(1), 77–91.

Yoder, P. J., Kaiser, A. P., Goldstein, H., Alpert, C., Mousetis, L., Kaczmarek, L., & Fischer, R. (1995). An exploratory comparison of milieu teaching and responsive interaction in classroom applications. *Journal of Early Intervention, 19*(3), 218–242. http://dx.doi.org/10.1177/105381519501900306

CHAPTER 2

Intervention as a Process

*AAC not only as an alternative means of communication
but a means to teach communication.*

—Dodd & Gorey, 2014

WHAT IS AN INTENSIVE, IMMERSIVE, SOCIALLY BASED AAC INTERVENTION?

The intervention model described in this book evolved through the author's experiences working with students with the most complex communication needs (CCNs), including those with significant cognitive impairments and severe autism. It was designed to target communication skills through the use of augmentative and alternative communication (AAC). The end goal is to support students with CCNs in achieving greater levels of communicative competence (ASHA, 2004; Light, 1989; Light & McNaughton, 2014). By utilizing natural interactions and experiences, and immersing the students in his or her AAC language, students accomplish much more. The intervention model described in this book enhances successful communication and minimizes social barriers (e.g., language gap) by providing training and support to communication partners and guides.

What Is an Intensive Intervention?

The most common service delivery model for students who are learning to communicate through the use of AAC is the traditional pull-out model. In this model, students receive a prescribed frequency (i.e., number of sessions per week) and duration (i.e., length of sessions) of services each week, usually individually, in an environment separate from their regular classroom. In fact, many parents that this author has encountered feel their child must have individual speech and language therapy provided in this format for their child to make progress. Once parents experience the progress their child is capable of making through their participation in the intervention model described in this book, they begin to recognize the benefits of an intervention model that is provided within real, authentic interactions. In this model, students receive the equivalent of a year's worth of speech-language services within a two-to-three-week time period. This allows students to firmly establish new skills before supports are faded. The problem with the traditional pull-out model, in which a student may be seen, for example, two to three times per week for sessions 20 to 30 minutes in length, is that a portion of each session must be devoted to re-teaching what was previously introduced several days earlier. These students need to practice newly introduced skills for them to become solidified. Additionally, at the end of the intense block of services, students return to their classroom with instructional staff who are also better trained in facilitating their communication skills within their daily routines. From this point, the speech-language pathologist may provide weekly lessons in the classroom or consultation. It is recommended that students receive 20 to 24 hours of intense intervention provided over the course of two or three weeks. This can be accomplished a variety of ways: for example, two hours daily for three weeks or three hours daily, Monday through Thursday for two weeks. The idea is for students to receive a block of intervention. Yes, this will require speech-language pathologists to be creative in the scheduling of these intense blocks of intervention. If school districts have an AAC specialist, this could be one way their time is applied at different sites throughout the district. Any opportunity to provide a more intense block of intervention will be most effective in meeting the needs of these students.

What Is an Immersive Intervention?

Consider how many times a typically developing child hears a target word such as "car" in context before they actually speak it. They usually experience this word multiple times by multiple communication partners before they attempt to say the word themselves. "Children learn to comprehend and produce words that are frequently spoken to them" (Harris & Reichle, 2004, p. 155). In fact, typically developing children acquire language by being immersed in the language they are learning. Now consider how many times a student, who is learning to communicate through the use of AAC, experiences the language of their communication system within context before being expected to use it. Unfortunately, for students who are expected to learn to communicate through the use of AAC, there is discrepancy between language exposure opportunities and AAC outcomes. There is a "mismatch" between exposure opportunities and expected outcomes. Input models (oral language) do not match output expectations (aided language) (Porter, 2007). Learning to communicate with AAC is similar to learning a second language; novice AAC users must be immersed in the language they are expected to acquire (Cafiero, 1998).

For students who are learning to communicate through AAC, immersion occurs when the facilitating adults use the same language system that the student is learning, and when the students are given opportunities to experience the symbols of their language in print, as visual supports, including adapted stories and visuals schedules. Adapted stories, a concept introduced by this author, are stories that have been modified physically, linguistically, and cognitively, so that they are manageable for students with CCNs. Chapter 4, *Intervention Planning Phase*, describes in detail the purpose of adapted stories and how to create them. Chapter 5, *Intervention Implementation Phase*, provides strategies for using them to facilitate language.

What Is a Socially Based Intervention?

A socially based intervention is one in which AAC skills are targeted through meaningful interactions. Students learn to use their communication systems while participating in activities that are motivating and engaging. Students experience the language of their communication systems in real context and are given opportunities to practice using them. A socially based intervention is one in which students learn to communicate within real contexts and is necessary in order to address all areas of communicative competence. A pull-out intervention model, as previously described, can be utilized to introduce skills in the areas of linguistic and operational competencies. However, in order for students to develop skills specific to social and strategic competencies, they must have opportunities to practice AAC use within real, authentic interactions (Table 2–1). Students who are motivated to communicate are more likely to practice learned skills in other contexts. Students learn that communication is an enjoyable experience that creates a means to an end. It is for these reasons that an effective AAC intervention is based on social interactions.

Table 2–1. Comparing Intervention Models

Pull-Out Model	*Intensive, Immersive, Social Model*
Linguistic Competence	Linguistic Competence
Operational Competence	Operational Competence
	Social Competence
	Strategic Competence

AAC INTERVENTION AS A PROCESS

Intervention, particularly as it relates to AAC, is a dynamic process—constantly shifting in response to a student's reaction to the intervention itself, and their changing communication needs. As a process, an AAC-based intervention is a series of deliberate steps taken to progress a student with complex communication needs (CCNs) toward greater levels of communicative competence (Schlosser, Koul, & Costello, 2007). However, it should not be viewed as a linear process in which first you do this, then you do this, and then you do this. Rather, in application, it is a fluid process in which there is constant shifting back and forth between steps as the student's skills and communication needs change. These intentional steps, referred to as phases, are based on and include activities related to assessment, intervention planning, and ultimately, implementation of the intervention (Schlosser et al.). Table 2–2 provides an overview of the different components at each phase of the intervention process. The subsequent sections will provide a detailed description of each component of the assessment, intervention planning, and the intervention implementation phases.

Assessment Phase

Assessment is the first phase of the intervention process. The purpose of an AAC evaluation is three-fold: (1) determine if a student would benefit from an AAC system; if so, (2) identify the appropriate AAC system based on the

Table 2–2. Phases of the AAC Intervention Process

Assessment	Intervention Planning	Intervention Implementation
Describe current means of communication	Identification of intervention needs	Provide an intensive block of intervention
Identify communication needs	Establish intervention targets	Create an immersive environment
Assess AAC-related skills	Develop or program communication system considering vocabulary selection, representation, and organization	Promote AAC use through socially engaging activities and interactions
Recommend AAC system	Preparing for intervention implementation	

student's abilities and communication needs, and (3) guide educational planning. AAC assessments differ from traditional assessments of speech and language skills. Traditional speech and language evaluations seek to determine if a speech and/or language delay or disorder exists, whereas AAC evaluations assume a student's difficulty with communicating is long term and they may benefit from the use of AAC to support their development of communication skills. Some AAC evaluations appear complicated. This book proposes an approach to conducting AAC evaluations—translating theory to practice—that school-based assessment teams will find effective in connecting students with CCNs to appropriate communication systems.

Assessment should be conceptualized in two phases: appraisal and diagnostic (Darley, 1991). During the appraisal phase, information is gathered so that informed decisions can be made during the diagnostic phase. The AAC evaluations can be broken down into four steps: (1) describe current means of communication, (2) identify communication needs, (3) assess AAC-related skills, and (4) recommend AAC system.

Describe Current Means of Communication

Understanding a student's current means of communication is necessary for identifying the gap between what they are currently capable of communicating and the communication demands of their environments. Appraisal of a student's speech, language, and communication skills is an integral component of the AAC assessment process. It provides a foundation that directly influences decisions regarding what type of AAC system will best meet the needs of the student, as well as how best to instruct the student in using their AAC system. Frequently, a referral or request for an AAC evaluation is the end result of a recent evaluation; therefore, conducting a comprehensive assessment of a student's speech, language, and communication skills is not always necessary if the SLP concludes the current evaluation is valid and reflective of the student's current communication skills. In the event that a full evaluation of a student's speech, language, and communication skills is warranted, skills should be assessed within two broad domains: language functioning (e.g., expressive and receptive language skills, which includes their understanding and use of semantics, syntax, and morphology) and social communicative functioning (e.g., pragmatics, joint attention, and social communicative behaviors—specifically social skills and play skills).

Identify Communication Needs

The next step of the AAC assessment process is to identify the communication needs of the potential AAC user. This is accomplished by comparing an individual's current means of communication to the communication demands of the various environments and activities in which she or he is expected to participate. Identifying the communication needs of the potential AAC user is a critical step of the assessment process. Not only will it guide the team in selecting the appropriate AAC system but, particularly for those who are the target of the intervention approach described in this book, influence how the AAC user will be taught to use their communication system. The "Communication Demands and Opportunities Inventory," developed by the author of this book and the "Social Networks Communication Inventory" (Blackstone & Hunt Berg, 2012) are both useful assessment tools that can be used to assist in identifying the communication needs of the student with CCNs.

Assess AAC-Related Skills

The final aspect of the appraisal piece of the assessment process is to examine skills related to AAC use. Prior to recommending a particular AAC system, it is important to document the student's proficiency in various AAC-related skills. Each communication system, technology- and non-technology-based, is composed of features that make it unique and customizable. Feature matching is a common technique used to "match" the ability and needs of the potential AAC user with the most appropriate AAC system, device, and/or techniques.

Additionally, there are a number of criterion-referenced tasks and checklists to assess and identify various AAC-related skills. While there are a few assessment tools geared toward assessing or documenting AAC abilities, evaluators will also rely on dynamic assessment as part of the evaluative process. In dynamic assessment, specific skills are assessed, instruction is provided to teach a specific skill or improve a present level of execution, and then the skill is retested. This test-teach-retest assessment procedure is useful in appraising a student's ability to acquire new skills and makes an estimate relative to their potential rate of learning, which is key to developing goals. Dynamic assessment is used to supplement standardized testing for those students whose significant cognitive disabilities render those types of assessments unreliable and is critical when assessing students with significant cognitive disabilities whose true abilities are not fully assessed using standardized tests.

Recommend AAC System

At the conclusion of the assessment process, and following trials with systematically selected systems, a recommendation is made for a communication system that matches the student's communication needs, as well as the potential AAC skills he or she may develop. This translation of data and information gathered during the appraisal phase into recommendations specific to both the AAC system and intervention development concludes the assessment phase. Ongoing assessment of the student as his or her abilities develop and communication needs change is continuously revisited throughout the intervention process.

Intervention Planning Phase

The intervention planning phase is when deliberate consideration is given to decisions regarding programming (e.g., for high-tech and low-tech communication systems) or creating (e.g., non-tech communication systems such as a communication board or book) the student's AAC system. Considerations include the initial set of vocabulary and how that vocabulary will be represented and organized. It is during the intervention planning phase that needs of the student are outlined and the corresponding goals developed. Additionally, during this phase, time is devoted to planning for implementation. This includes strategies to engineer the environment so that learning can be supported. This time is set aside to train those who will be working with the student, or those will come into direct contact with the student on a regular basis.

Identify Intervention Needs

The intervention-planning phase begins by delineating the intervention needs of the student. This begins by understanding the student's current level of skills related to communication and AAC use, and utilizing the information assembled during the assessment phase. In principle, it is recognizing the student's current level of functioning and potential rate of learning based on how he or she responds during dynamic assessments. This is where dynamic assessment becomes directly linked to intervention implementation.

Establish Intervention Targets

Once a student's intervention needs are determined, the intervention team can move forward with developing goals and objectives to progress the student to greater levels of communicative competence. As will be repeatedly highlighted throughout this book, the overarching goal is to improve the student's communicative competence, and, therefore, goals need to be developed in each of the four competency areas. How to do this is covered in detail in Chapter 4, *Intervention Planning Phase* and Chapter 6, *Progress Monitoring*.

Program or Develop AAC System

Prior to implementing an AAC-based intervention, careful consideration should be given to not only the type of communication system being recommended, but how that system will be programmed. This holds true not only for students who will be using high-tech communication systems, but also for those students who will be using low-tech and non-tech communication systems. This is why so many intervention teams fail! So much attention is given to the technical aspects of programming, with very little forethought as to how the communication system should be developed or programmed, in order to facilitate communication and AAC use. It has been the author's experience that many teams just want to know how to add symbols or words, not to truly understanding the complexities of language. Of particular importance is determining which vocabulary will be represented on the student's communication system, and how those words will be organized and represented. Chapter 4, *Intervention Planning Phase*, provides a complete discussion regarding these concerns and many more, related to programming or creating a student's communication system.

Preparing for Implementation

The final aspect of the intervention-planning phase is to prepare for the actual implementation of the intervention. The focus is to create a language-rich environment. This can be accomplished by training communication guides in techniques and strategies to facilitate communication, such as with visual supports.

Engineer the Environment. A language-rich environment provides students with multiple opportunities to experience their AAC language throughout the course of their day. This can be accomplished by incorporating picture schedules, choice boards, adapted stories (Dodd, 2011), and the use of modeling boards. Adapted stories are stories that have been adapted or modified physically, linguistically, and cognitively for students with CCNs. Chapter 4 outlines how to create these adapted stories and Chapter 5 provides suggestions for using adapted stories during shared reading experiences in order to facilitate language and communication in children with CCNs.

Train Communication Guides. The last step of the intervention-planning phase involves training key participants. It is important that all participants understand the premise behind teaching certain words over others. This will be a paradigm shift for many. Many individuals who work with students with CCNs think that if the child is requesting preferred food items and reinforcers, requesting a break, or to use the restroom, they are communicating. Communication is much more dynamic than fulfilling immediate want and needs. In addition to learning the complexities of language, communication guides will learn how to apply familiar language-stimulation techniques (e.g., self-talk, modeling) to AAC through the use of aided modeling techniques (Table 2–3). This will contribute to creating the language rich environment we are striving for.

Intervention Implementation Phase

This is where we put it all into practice! Recall the primary objective is to promote the student with CCNs to a higher level of communicative compe-

Table 2–3. Language Stimulation Techniques Translated to AAC Intervention

Strategy	Definition	Application to AAC
Self-talk	Clinician describes his or her own actions as he or she engages in parallel play with child.	Communication guide pairs self-talk with ALgS to reinforce use of the targeted device.
Parallel-talk	Clinician provides a running description of the child's actions.	Running description is provided utilizing ALgS. This strategy provides a model for the child to internalize.
Modeling	Clinician provides an example of target production.	Communication guide provides an example of a novel, meaningful production using the targeted AAC device.
Expansion	Clinician repeats child's utterance with an additional word or phrase, which creates a more semantically or syntactically complete utterance.	Communication guide repeats child's production and adds symbols to the child's initial message to create a more syntactically complete message.

Source: Dodd, & Gorey, 2014. Printed with permission.

tence. Guiding the student in accessing his or her communication system and empowering them to create novel messages for a variety of functions leads the child towards independent, participatory communication. This is accomplished by immersing the child in an environment rich in AAC language, while simultaneously creating opportunities for using his or her communication system. An effective AAC intervention is intensive, immersive, and social.

Provide Intensive Block of Intervention

Intervention intensity is typically based on a number of variables including (1) form (e.g., drill, play), (2) dose (e.g., number of trials), (3) duration (i.e., length of session), (4) frequency (e.g., number of sessions per week), (5) total intervention time (e.g., number of times), and (6) cumulative intervention intensity (i.e., total number of practice opportunities over time) (Warren, Fey, & Yoder, 2007). Preliminary research (Dodd & Hagge, 2014) related to the intervention described in this book suggests a positive correlation between an intense block of intervention and students' progress. As previously stated in this chapter, a block of intervention, such as 20 to 26 hours, provided over the course of two to three weeks is necessary in order to firmly establish new skills.

Create an Immersive Environment

As previously discussed in this chapter, children learn language by being immersed in the language they are attempting to learn. Therefore, for this intervention to be effective, the student must be immersed in the language of their communication system. Several suggestions of how this is accomplished are presented in this chapter and is discussed throughout this book.

Promote AAC Use Through Socially Engaging Activities

In the end, the activities selected for teaching students how to communicate through the use of AAC should be socially engaging. To experience the value of communication, students should have varied and multiple opportunities to practice. "Communication" is not a static process; it is a fluid, dynamic process that students must practice within real contexts. Optimally, the student benefits by learning to practice "communication" authentically, in real learning experiences and contexts.

The intensive, immersive, and socially based intervention model discussed throughout this book elevates students to greater levels of communicative competence.

REFERENCES

American Speech-Language Hearing Association (ASHA). (2004). *Roles and responsibilities of speech-language pathologists with respect to augmentative and alternative communication. Technical report.* Retrieved from http://www.asha.org/policy/TR 2004-00262/

Blackstone, S., & Hunt Berg, M. (2012). *Social networks: A communication inventory for individuals with complex communication needs and their communication partners, revised version.* Verona, WI: Attainment.

Cafiero, J. (1998). Communication power for individuals with autism. *Focus on Autism and Other Developmental Disabilities, 13,* 113–121.

Darley, F. (1991). A philosophy of appraisal and diagnosis. In F. Darley & D. Spriestersbach (Eds.), *Diagnostic methods in speech pathology* (22nd ed., pp. 1–23). Prospect Height, IL: Waveland Press.

Dodd, J. L. (2011). Creating early literacy opportunities for children with complex communication needs. In M. F. Shaughnessy & K. Kleyn (Eds.), *Handbook of early childhood education.* Hauppauge, NY: Nova Science.

Dodd, J. L., & Gorey, M. (2014). AAC intervention as an immersion model. *Communication Disorders Quarterly, 35*(2), 103–107. http://dx.doi.org/10.1177/1525740113504242

Dodd, J. L., & Hagge, D. (2014). AAC camp as an alternative school based service delivery model: A retrospective survey. *Communication Disorders Quarterly, 35*(3), 123–132. http://dx.doi.org/10.1177/1525740113512670

Harris, M., & Reichle, J. (2004). The impact of aided language stimulation on symbol comprehension and production in children with moderate cognitive disabilities. *American Journal of Speech-Language Pathology, 13,* 155–167.

Light, J. (1989). Toward a definition of communicative competence for individuals using augmentative and alternative communication systems. *Augmentative and Alternative Communication, 5*(2), 137–144.

Light, J., & McNaughton, D. (2014). Communicative competence for individuals who require augmentative and alternative communication: A new definition for a new era of communication? *Augmentative and Alternative Communication, 30*(1), 1–18.

Porter, G. (2007). *PODDs: Pragmatically organized dynamic displays.* Melbourne, Australia: Cerebral Palsy Education Centre & Communication Resource Centre.

Schlosser, R. W., Koul, R., & Costello, J. (2007). Asking well-built questions for evidence-based practice in augmentative and alternative communication. *Journal of Communication Disorders, 40,* 225–238.

Warren, S. F., Fey, M. E., & Yoder, P. J. (2007). Differential treatment intensity research: A missing link to creating optimally effective communication interventions. *Mental Retardation and Developmental Disabilities Research Reviews, 13*(1), 70–77.

CHAPTER 3

Assessment Phase

Assessment is a necessary piece of the intervention process. A comprehensive AAC evaluation is the foundation of a deliberately framed intervention program. It is a multifaceted problem-solving process that involves collecting information about a student from a multitude of resources. The data, which are methodically collected and interpreted, are used to make informed decisions that will impact a student's movement toward greater levels of communicative competence. An AAC evaluation, as a process, enables invested stakeholders to understand the current communication abilities and needs of the individual so that a plan can be devised to assist that student in becoming an active participant in his or her environment.

Assessment can be conceptualized in two phases: the appraisal phase and the diagnostic phase (Darley, 1991). During the appraisal phase, relevant data is compiled from different resources, including a student's case history, interviews with parents and other professionals, review of school and medical records, and evaluation by the clinician (Darley). The studying and interpretation of the data for guiding therapeutic decisions encapsulates the diagnostic phase. By dedicating time to the assessment process, intervention teams form the foundation from which to develop a comprehensive intervention program.

How do AAC evaluations differ from other types of educationally relevant assessments? According to Quill, Bracken, and Fair (2000), an "educational assessment of children serves three basic purposes: to provide an estimate of developmental functioning, to describe skills needed for planning intervention, and to document development and progress over time" (p. 39). Unlike traditional speech and language evaluations in which the purpose is to determine if a disability or disorder exists and if the student "qualifies" for special education services, AAC evaluations acknowledge that a delay or disorder exists and are pursued for the purpose of helping an individual gain greater access to communication. The end result of an AAC evaluation is to guide the intervention process, including identifying an appropriate AAC system and strategies to help the student. The purpose of assessment, as it relates to AAC, is threefold. First, it determines if a student would benefit from an AAC system. Any student who is nonverbal or unable to effectively communicate using oral language is a candidate for AAC. AAC encompasses a wide range of communication options, including technology- and non-technology-based systems. The second purpose is to compile information so that the appropriate AAC system can be selected and/or devised. The final purpose of an AAC evaluation is to guide intervention teams in developing an educational plan to support the student's acquisition of communication. In the end, an AAC evaluation contributes to the selection of a communication system, and guides intervention planning and intervention implementation.

AAC EVALUATION AS A NECESSARY STEP

Unfortunately, it has become common practice for teams to introduce a student to an AAC system, generally AAC apps, exclusive of an AAC evaluation. The reasons this occurs are numerous, some of which are understandable, but it is not considered best practices to recommend an AAC system without a formal AAC evaluation, not to mention that it could be considered a violation of a free and appropriated education (FAPE) (IDEA, 2004). An AAC evaluation is more than just an assessment; it is an opportunity to understand the expectations of involved parties with regard to why they are seeking an AAC system for their child or student. It is an opportunity to begin to teach those working with the student to the benefits and limitations of an AAC system, and what it takes in order for a student to be a successful AAC user. Too often, AAC apps are purchased and then the speech-language pathologist (SLP) is brought in afterward to problem solve why it isn't working. The SLP is expected to understand the purposes for which the AAC system was recommended in the first place. This is backward and will surely impede the student's success in using their AAC system. The best way to support parents and families is to recognize their desired outcomes and let them know what skills need to be first developed to progress a child toward that level of competency. Many of the assessment tools suggested throughout this chapter can assist parents in recognizing the precursor skills that support their child's achievement of desired outcomes.

An AAC evaluation does not begin with looking at which communication aid the student needs. It begins by looking at the current communication skills of the individual and the disparity between those skills and what it is that the student needs to communicate. The barriers that may potentially impede their access to communication can be identified and partially addressed during the assessment process. It is during this time that benefits, limitations, and options are revealed and discussed with parents and interested parties. It is also an opportunity to answer questions and clear up any preconceived thoughts or misconceptions that may exist.

A MODEL OF ASSESSMENT TO SUPPORT INTERVENTION

The Participation Model (Beukelman & Mirenda, 2013) provides a framework for conducting AAC evaluations and implementing related interventions (ASHA, 2004). The Participation Model begins with identifying the individual's participation patterns and communication needs. This is established by observing the student within regularly occurring activities and environments, then comparing the targeted student's ability to participate in these activities relative to the participation patterns of their peers. From there, barriers to their participation to a level commensurate with their peers are identified. Barriers, as they relate to AAC, includes something or someone that make it difficult or impossible, or prevents, hinders, or blocks, a person from participating in or accessing activities to an equivalent level of competency as their peers. Based on Beukelman and Mirenda's Participation Model, barriers are considered with relation to access and opportunity.

Access Barriers

As described by Beukelman and Mirenda (2013), access barriers "pertain to the capabilities, attitudes, and resource limitations of people who communicate through AAC" (p. 116). Identification of access barriers begins with having a comprehensive understanding of the student's current communication abilities. Within this area of assessment, the student's potential to improve or increase their ability to use natural speech is gauged, their ability to benefit from environmental adaptations is considered, and their skills related to utilizing an AAC communication system are appraised.

Opportunity Barriers

Opportunity barriers can be classified into one of the five categories: policy, practice, knowledge, skill, and attitude. Inevitably, opportunity barriers will exist; however, the manner in which we respond to these barriers will influence the success of our students' access to communication. Some barriers will be addressed through training and educating interested parties, others will require us to navigate around, and others will require us to just to continue to press forward.

Policy and practice barriers, which are frequently referred to synonymously when in fact they are distinctly different, can impede a student's success in using their AAC system. Policy barriers refer to formal regulatory or legislative procedures that govern the environments and organizations many students with CCNs participate in regularly (e.g., schools, extracurricular activities such as clubs and sport teams). With the Individuals with

Disabilities Education Act (IDEA, 2004) and the reauthorization of No Child Left Behind (NCLB, 2001), and the Every Student Succeeds Act (ESSA, 2015), these types of barriers are diminishing in certain environments, giving students who use AAC greater access to typically developing peers and the technologies they need. It is perhaps practice barriers, actions that are common among members of an organization which are mistakenly believing these common procedures are in fact policies that they must adhere to, that pose the greatest challenge to students with CCNs. The next three categories of barriers are to a degree intertwined, spreading and influencing the other. Knowledge, skill, and attitude barriers all have the potential to block an emergent communicator's access to AAC. Ideally, through educating and training those involved, we can improve skills and change attitudes.

OVERVIEW OF ASSESSMENT

Unlike traditional speech and language evaluations that report specific scores related to students' performance on specific standardized tests, AAC evaluations reflect a gathering of information for purposes of identifying a student's current levels of performance, and determining how an ACC system or strategies can support their communication efforts. Dynamic assessment and use of standardized assessment are the most common types of assessment tools used when assessing speech and language skills in young children. Dynamic assessment is an assessment strategy in which a skill or skills identified as a challenge during assessment are targeted briefly, and then reassessed to gain insight to a child's or student's learning potential (ASHA, 2016). This test-teach-test approach is often used to distinguish between a language difference and a language disorder, and is also often used in conjunction with standardized assessments and language sampling. More specifically, with respect to AAC evaluations, gaining insight into a student's learning potential informs intervention planning, allowing intervention teams to make predictions about how a student might respond to a particular intervention over a specified period of time. Table 3–1 describes standardized assessments, which are typically used with respect to assessing language, communication, and AAC-related skills.

Age Appropriate Versus Developmentally Appropriate

Students with CNNs present with significant delays with respect to communication and language, in comparison to typically developing age-matched peers. The challenge is that giving this group of students tests designed and developed for students of the same age or grade may not always be the best tools for identifying their strengths and weaknesses. A test that tells you the student is performing below the first percentile provides you with very

Table 3–1. Two Types of Standardized Assessment Tools

Standardized Assessments

Standardized assessments refer to any test that is administered and scored in a "standard" or consistent manner. Standardized tests require all examinees to answer the same questions or items in a prescribed manner, making it possible to compare their performance to other test takers or groups of test takers who took the same test. There are two types of standardized assessment tools, and these are criterion-referenced and norm-referenced.

Criterion-Referenced	***Norm-Referenced***
Criterion-referenced tests are standardized tests that evaluate an individual's performance relative to predetermined criteria or performance standards. They are used to determine if an individual has achieved specific skills. An individual's performance is compared to a preset standard regardless of the performance of other test takers. Criterion-referenced tests are useful in identifying a student's present level of performance in target areas and the results can be used for instructional planning purposes (e.g., descriptions of what an individual is expected to know or be able to do at a specific stage of development or level of education). In educational settings, criterion-referenced tests may be used to assess whether the student has learned a specific body of knowledge. It is possible, and in fact desirable, for an individual to pass or earn a perfect score on a criterion-referenced test.	Norm-referenced tests are standardized tests specifically developed to rank test takers comparatively to age- or grade-level matched peers. Based on their performance, test takers are ranked according to a bell curve. A bell curve distribution is characterized by a small percentage of individuals performing either very well or above the average or below the average range, with a majority of test takers performing within the "average range." Performance on norm-referenced tests is typically reported as a percentage or percentile rank. For example, a student whose performance equates to a 75th percentile ranking is considered to have performed as well as or better than 75% of those who took the same test, with 25% of test takers performing better.

Sources: ASHA, 2016; Hidden Curriculum, 2014; Popham, 1975.

little information from which to help support the child. It only tells you the student is severely impaired (you already knew that). In these instances, it is important to select assessment tools that are developmentally appropriate, as opposed to age appropriate. In fact, some standardized assessment tools state the test is for a prescribed age range (e.g., children two to five years of age) or for someone functioning within that age range (e.g., PLS-5). In the event you select to use these more developmentally appropriate assessment tools, you obviously cannot report standardized test scores because the student is outside of the normative data. Reporting age equivalency scores is further discouraged as there are inherent psychometric problems with translating raw scores into age-equivalency scores. It is suggested to use the information for descriptive purposes and establishing baseline performances only. The information acquired from standardized tests is invaluable and should be incorporated whenever appropriate.

AAC EVALUATION: FROM THEORY TO PRACTICE

In the beginning of this chapter, Beukelman and Mirenda's Participation Model (2013), which is supported by the American Speech-Language Hearing Association (ASHA) (2004) as the preferred framework for conducting AAC evaluations and implementing related interventions, was introduced. The remainder of this chapter will present how to implement this model from theory to practice. Specifically, how school-based assessment teams can implement a Participation Model-based assessment. In the event a school-based assessment team is seeking funding from an external source such as Medi-Cal or private insurance, the team will want to refer to those organizations for specifics in submitting their findings. The information acquired through the procedures described here can be easily aligned with the requirements of these particular agencies.

An AAC evaluation can be conceptualized as a four-step process in which the team begins by understanding the student's current means of communication and how that compares to the communication demands of their environment. Then AAC-related skills are assessed, and recommendations to the type of AAC system and the strategies that are best suited to meet the needs of the individual are outlined. It is suggested that assessment findings be reported using the following headings: reason for referral, background information, current means of communication, identification of communication needs, and recommendations. The remainder of the chapter discusses how to gather and report information in each of these areas and provides an overview of tools and procedures that can be used.

AAC evaluation is a four-step process:

✓ Identify student's current means of communication.

✓ Identify communication needs.

✓ Assess AAC-related skills.

✓ Recommend AAC system and intervention supports and strategies.

Reason for Referral

At the onset of the assessment process it is important to understand the reason(s) a family or intervention team is pursuing an assessment. What is it the family or team hopes to accomplish at the end of this process? This is a necessary step because it will help you understand the family or team's perspective and expectations of what an AAC system can do for their child or student. For example, consider a five year-old child whose speech is severely unintelligible. It has been determined that the probability of this individual developing intelligible speech is highly unlikely due to a combination of respiratory challenges, facial anomalies, and facial paralysis. The child is verbal and her parents understand most of what she says when the context is known. However, it is extremely difficult to understand the content of her communication attempts when the context is unknown, and for those less familiar with her speech patterns, it becomes exponentially more difficult to understand her speech. Her current speech-language pathologist estimates that she is using four-to-five-word sentences, but this is only an approximation due to her highly unintelligible speech. The five-year-old little girl is currently employing a variety of strategies to compensate for her unintelligible speech, including the use of gestures and descriptive language to help her communication partners understand the content of her messages. She is getting ready to enter a general education kindergarten and her parents want an AAC system she can use when she is not understood by her peers or teacher. Preliminarily, this child appears to be an ideal candidate for a high-tech communication system that will allow her to create syntactically and morphologically correct sentences. The challenge is that this type of system requires the AAC user to use it on a regular basis in order for them to become fluid in their communication. With only occasional use of an AAC system of this complexity, it will be difficult for this child to become proficient. Therefore, throughout the assessment process, it will be important to support the family in understanding what it takes to become a proficient AAC user. Furthermore, the team may want to explore other augmentative strategies (e.g., remnant book or topic board) to enhance the listener's understanding of the little girl's communication attempts.

A **remnant book** is a small photo album that AAC users employ to store remnants of recent activities (e.g., movie stub, amusement park wristband). These remnants allow the individual to share recent experiences by giving their communication partners a clue to the topic of conversation. **Topic boards** that are composed of "preferred topics of conversation" serve a similar function. Narrowing the topic of conversation to a specific topic gives a context to support their listener's comprehension of their speech (Beukelman & Mirenda, 2013).

Contrastively, consider the parent of a child with severe autism may feel an AAC system will finally help their child communicate. You recognize that the child has difficulty with pre-linguistic skills such as communicative intent and joint attention. As you progress through the assessment process, you can begin to assist the family in understanding the scope of their child's communication disability and the precursor skills necessary for successful communication to occur. Note that I did not say "precursor skills necessary for AAC use." An AAC system can be used to teach these precursor communication skills.

When conducting an AAC evaluation it is imperative to consider the preferences and desires of those involved, help those participants understand what it takes to use a complex AAC system, and identify intervention strategies that will support the student in achieving greater levels of communicative competence.

Background Information

In order to develop a detailed understanding of the student's current abilities, both in communication skills and AAC-related skills, start the assessment process by reviewing pertinent background information. Background information, in part, can be compiled by reviewing previous assessment reports and other relevant paperwork contained within a student's confidential file. A student's confidential file, which may be kept at their school or in a central administrative office (e.g., special education administrative office), contains assessment reports including, initial assessments for consideration of eligibility for special education services and subsequent triennial assessments, along with reports that may have been conducted by independent evaluators. Also, within the confidential file are medical records that have been released, student's Individualized Education Programs (IEPs) and, often, correspondences between parents and school personnel. Unlike cumulative files, access to confidential files is limited and granted only to certain individuals. In addition to reviewing previous assessment reports and IEPs, it is essential to interview parents. It is quite probable that information previously reported has changed, or perhaps reported inaccurately. In addition to gathering information from a parent interview and review of other related documents, additional insight to these key areas will be observed throughout the assessment process. When gathering background information, specifically as it relates to an AAC evaluation, it is necessary to assemble information regarding the student in the following areas: medical history, visual and hearing status, mobility status, educational history, and cognitive status.

Medical History

Many children with CCNs have equally complicating medical histories. It is not uncommon for these children to have been the product of a complicated pregnancy and/or birth and, thus, present with developmental challenges that are frequently noted early in the child's development. Children with CCNs may present with histories of digestive issues and/or food allergies, among other medical complications. Understanding what medications they have taken or are currently taking is helpful in further understanding the complexities of their condition(s). Many medications can have a positive or negative effect on the overall alertness of the individual, and can affect their overall demeanor. When taking a medical history, be sure to note any food allergies or aversions. Are they on a special diet? Children may be on a gluten-free diet. Always note the reason(s) for specialized diets or food restrictions (e.g., to assist in controlling seizures). Have they had any surgeries? If so, note when and for what reason, as well as the outcome. A comprehensive medical history is imperative in understanding the influencing factors on the student's communication skills.

Visual and Hearing Status

Hearing and visual acuity is routinely assessed as part of a student's initial or triennial assessment. Students who receive special education services must be re-evaluated every three years to determine if they continue to need special education services (Moore & Montgomery, 2016). As an element of these multidisciplinary assessments, vision and hearing at a minimum is screened. In the event the individual being assessed does not have a current vision or hearing screening or evaluation (or you feel they are in need of a more in-depth assessment) you will want to make the appropriate referral. If there are concerns related to hearing or vision it is, important to identify them early in the AAC assessment process. Many students with CCNs can be hard to assess using traditional assessment procedures, so having someone who is skilled in assessing individuals who are nonverbal or with multiple disabilities is preferred.

A student's vision abilities will have direct implications on the type (e.g., real photos, black/white or colored icons), size, and placement of icons. The following are examples of questions a skilled vision specialist may ask a parent in order to gain a better sense of their child's vision abilities:

- ◆ Does your child smile when a parent comes up to her? (assesses near vision)
- ◆ Does your child smile when a parent enters the room? (assesses distance vision)
- ◆ Does your child blink or close his eyes when a light is turned on or he is brought outside? (response to light)
- ◆ Does your child see herself or himself in the mirror and respond (reaching toward mirror, vocalizing, etc.)? (assesses near vision)
- ◆ Does your child reach for an object placed in front of him or her? (assesses near vision)

◆ If the lights are turned off, does your child respond? (assesses response to light)
◆ Does your child blink when a hand is moved in front of or toward his face? (blink reflex)
◆ Does your child pick up a toy or piece of food and put it in her or his mouth? (assesses near vision)
◆ Does your child imitate facial expressions? (assesses distance vision).

Unfortunately, these types of questions also tap into the core deficits of many children with CCNs. It is possible that a student with CCNs may appear to exhibit vision challenges, when in fact their failed responses are influenced by the core deficits of their diagnosis. For example, consider a child who has difficulty with *line of regard*. Line of regard refers to a child's ability to follow an adult's gaze in anticipation that there will be an event of shared interest (Johnston, Reichle, Feeley, & Jones, 2012). This same child may have difficulty with imitation in general, not just imitation of facial gestures. Children with autism are not always responsive to those in their immediate environment, which may make it appear as though they have deficiencies in their vision. So the potential for false positive is quite possible. Contrastively, the inverse conclusion may also be drawn and vision deficits are often missed as well.

Although it does not have direct implications as to symbol size and location of symbols, hearing is another area of assessment that should be current and accurate. It may affect the type of voice output you select and loudness, and overall how you approach teaching communication to the student with CCNs.

Mobility Status

In this section, the student's ambulatory or non-ambulatory status is identified. An individual who is considered ambulatory is capable of walking independently without the assistance of another person or adaptive equipment (e.g., wheelchair, walker). Those who are identified as non-ambulatory are dependent on the assistance of another person, walker, or wheelchair. As it relates to AAC, it necessary to know if the individual can independently locate and retrieve their AAC system. The team may need to consider teaching strategies to increase the individual's independent access (operational competence) of their communication system to the maximum extent possible, taking into consideration their physical constraints. A detailed evaluation of the potential AAC user's physical capabilities may be warranted when you conduct your *Capability Assessment*.

Educational History

By reviewing the student's educational history, you will gain insight to what interventions have been attempted, as well as the student's success with those interventions. It is necessary to review what types of support services the student has received over the years and how those services have changed. What types(s) of school experiences has the student had? It is possible that a student has received an extensive amount of early intervention services beginning at an early age, or that, perhaps, this is their first school experience. All these experiences (or lack thereof) will have an impact on the student's readiness for an AAC system. This information will help decide what types of supports need to be in place to ensure the student is successful in using their AAC system.

Another interesting informative aspect of a student's history is to review previous individualized educational programs (IEPs). It is not uncommon for older students who continue to be bereft of functional communication skills to experience what the authors refer to as "Goal Recyclement." Goal Recyclement occurs when a student appears to recycle through goals every few years. For example, a student may have been exposed to Picture Exchange Communication System (PECS) at a young age. For one reason or another, the approach was abandoned and a different approach to teaching communication (e.g., Functional Communication Training) was introduced. After a few years of trying various other treatment approaches with varying degrees of success, PECS is reintroduced and the cycle begins again. Unfortunately, this recycling phenomenon occurs for a multitude of reasons. One reason may be differing perspectives on the best method to teaching a student with CCNs to communicate. As a student matriculates through the educational system, and moves from one class to another, one school to another, or from one program to another, different intervention teams have differing views of what methods they feel is best to address the needs of the student. Another potential influence may be in response to the perception that the student is not making progress or they are not making progress fast enough. Intervention teams may feel pressure to try something different when progress is not easily recognized. Many students with CCNs do progress at a slower rate, and their successes are not easily measured utilizing current approaches. Some intervention teams are disinclined to consider alternative approaches because they do not have the experience or comfort level with the intervention being implemented. Right or wrong, these are real reasons why intervention approaches are abandoned, news ones introduced, and previously abolished approaches reintroduced.

Cognitive Status

Although not necessarily formally assessed as a component of the AAC evaluation, an assessment team should be prepared to report on a student's cognitive abilities as they relate to AAC use. As discussed in Chapter 1, there is no prerequisite level of cognition that determines if an individual is a candidate for an AAC system. However, understanding an individual's strengths and weaknesses guides a team in developing a comprehensive intervention plan. This will include not only what AAC system to recommend, but also the strategies to assist the AAC user in learning to communicate.

As demonstrated, assembling critical background information is the first step in identifying potential barriers that may hinder an individual's *access* to an AAC system, and those potential *opportunity* barriers that may already exist.

Assessment

As previously stated, an AAC assessment is less about administering a battery of tests than a process of gathering information so informed decisions can be made. The actual "assessment" piece involves, if necessary, administration of standardized tests, but more importantly, assembling of information in order to describe a student's abilities in three key areas: current means of communication, communication needs, and AAC-related skills.

Identify Student's Current Means of Communication

Appraisal of a student's speech, language, and communication skills is an important component of the AAC assessment process. This provides a foundation that directly influences decisions regarding what type of AAC system will best meet the needs of the student, and how to instruct the student in using their AAC system. Frequently, referral for AAC evaluations is the end result of a recent evaluation; therefore, conducting a comprehensive assessment of a student's speech, language, and communication skills may not be necessary if the AAC evaluation team feels the information from recent testing is valid and reflective of the student's current abilities. In the event there is not a recent comprehensive assessment or critical elements are missing from that evaluation, a comprehensive evalution of the student's speech, language, and communication skills will be necessary.

In the event a full evaluation of a student's speech, language and communication skills is necessary, skills should be assessed within two broad domains: language functioning and social communicative functioning. Language functioning refers to the student's overall expressive and receptive language skills, which includes their understanding and use of semantics, syntax, and morphology. With regard to social communicative functioning, skills are examined in the areas of pragmatics, joint attention, and social communicative behaviors—specifically social skills and play skills. Table 3–2 provides an overview of various assessment tools that may be considered in assessing these areas of functioning. It is necessary to remember that children with complex communication needs do not always communicate via conventional means. Oftentimes, their means of communication are not easily or sufficiently documented using traditional assessments protocols. Therefore, it is recommended that assessment teams implement a wide range of assessment tools when evaluating language and communication skills in this particular group of students.

Table 3–2. Assessing Language and Social Communicative Functioning in Students with CCNs

Language Functioning	
Semantic Knowledge	MacArthur-Bates Communicative Development Inventories (MCDI) (Fenson, Marchman, Thal, Dale, Reznick, & Bates, 2006)
Expressive Language Skills	Inventory of Communicative Means
	Language Sample
Receptive Language Skills	Test of Auditory Comprehension of Language, 4th Edition (TACL-4) (Carrow-Woolfolk, 2014)
	Inventory of Semantic Relations
	Inventory of Wh-questions
Overall Language Skills	Rossetti Infant Toddler Scale (Rossetti, 2006)
	Preschool Language Scales, 5th Edition (PLS-5) (Zimmerman, Steiner, & Pond, 2011)
	Functional Communication Profile, Revised Edition (FCP-R) (Kleiman, 2003)
	SCERTS Assessment Process (SAP): Social Partner and Language Partner Stages-*Symbol Use* (Prizant, Wetherby, Rubin, Laurent, & Rydell, 2006)
Social Communicative Functioning	
Pragmatics	Inventory of Communicative Functions
	Communication and Symbolic Behavior Scales Developmental Profile (CSBS:DP) (Wetherby & Prizant, 2002)
	The Communication Matrix (Rowland, 2016)
Social Cognition	SCERTS Assessment Process (SAP): Social Partner and Language Partner Stages-*Joint Attention* (Prizant, Wetherby, Rubin, Laurent, & Rydell, 2006)
Social Communicative Behaviors	*Social Skills*—Social Skills Checklist (Quill, Bracken, & Fair, 2000)
	Play Skills—Developmental Playscale (Westby, 2000)

Sources: Dodd, 2010; Dodd, Franke, Grzesik, & Stoskopf, 2014.

Assessment Tools and Strategies

MacArthur-Bates Communicative Development Inventory: Words and Gestures. The MacArthur-Bates Communicative Development Inventory:

Words and Gestures (MCDI) (Fenson et al., 2006). utilizes parents as informants in reporting their child's first nonverbal gestural signals, their understanding and use of vocabulary, and early grammatical forms. It will take parents approximately 20 to 40 minutes to complete, and then the clinician, an additional 10 to 15 minutes to score. Parents report on their child's initial understanding of oral language (e.g., respond to their name. cease an action in response to hearing, "no-no"), along with key phrases and familiar requests (e.g., "Are you hungry?" "Throw the ball."). Subsequently, the parents are given a comprehensive inventory of vocabulary terms grouped by familiar categories (e.g., animals, toys, clothing), and asked to identify those terms their child "understands," and those vocabulary items their child "understands and says." In the end, the professional has a comprehensive inventory of the words the child knows and uses.

Rossetti Infant Toddler Scale™. The Rossetti Infant-Toddler Language Scale (Rossetti, 2006) is a criterion-referenced checklist that can be used to identify preverbal and verbal aspects of communication in infants to three years of age. The checklist is divided into six subtests: Interaction-Attachment, Pragmatics, Gesture, Play, Language Comprehension, and Language Expression. Behaviors can be directly elicited from the child or reported by the parent, all of which are considered equally a valid means of data collection. The following provides a brief summary of each subtest:

- Interaction Attachment: This subtest assesses the cues and responses exhibited by the child that reflect a reciprocal relationship between the caregiver and the child.
- Pragmatics: This subtest examines the way the child uses language to communicate with and affect others in a social manner.
- Gesture: This subtest assesses the child's use of gestures to express thoughts and intent prior to the consistent use of spoken language.
- Play: This subtest records changes in a child's play that reflect the development of representational thought.
- Language Comprehension: This subtest assesses the child's understanding of verbal language with and without linguistic cues.
- Language Expression: This subtest assesses the child's use of preverbal and verbal behaviors to communicate with others.

Preschool Language Scales, 5th Edition (PLS-5). The Preschool Language Scales, 5th Edition (PLS-5) (Zimmerman, Steiner, & Pont, 2011) is a norm-referenced assessment of developmental language skills. Although it was developed for children between birth to seven years, 11 months of age, it can be used with older students who are functioning within this age range. The PLS-5 can be used to assist in differentiating the presence of a language delay versus a language disorder. It can assess if the child is experiencing difficulties in the receptive or expressive aspects of language or if they are experiencing dual difficulties. In addition to providing a Total Language Score, the PLS-5 yields both an Auditory Comprehension (AC) and Expressive Communication (EC) scores. The Auditory Comprehension scale evaluates a child's understanding of language, including their knowledge of vocabulary, basic concepts, morphology, and syntax. Used with older children, it assesses understanding of complex sentences, inferential thinking, and emergent literacy skills. The Expressive Communication scale evaluates a child's ability to describe objects, use various morphological structures, use prepositions to describe object locations, and express comparisons and inferences. The PLS-5 is useful not only in identifying a child's strengths and weaknesses, but also as a means to evaluate a student's response to treatment.

Functional Communication Profile™, Revised. The Functional Communication Profile, Revised Edition (FCP-R) (Kleinman, 2003) provides an overall inventory of an individual's communication abilities, including their preferred mode of communication (e.g., verbal, sign, nonverbal, augmentative), and level of independence in executing specific skills. Individuals who present with mild to profound deficits are assessed and rated in the major skill categories of communication through direct observation, teacher and caregiver reports, and one-on-one testing. This assessment tool provides a detailed overview of a student's language skills, with attention given to examining their pragmatic and social use of language, beginning with the foundational skills of communicative intent and initiation. With reference to expressive language skills, there is an opportunity to create an inventory of basic communication skills, including both symbolic and non-symbolic forms of communication related to expressing preferences and pleasure or discomfort, and to labeling objects within their immediate environment. The following provides an overview of the different subtests and skills examined within each subtest:

- Sensory/Motor assesses a student's auditory, visual, gross-motor, and fine-motor skills and behaviors.
- Attentiveness assesses a student's attention span, alertness, response levels, cooperation, and level of awareness.
- Receptive Language assess a student's comprehension of verbal and nonverbal language and basic concepts, interest in pictures and objects, ability to follow commands, and recognition of objects and two-dimensional pictures.
- Expressive Language assesses a student's verbal and nonverbal communication skills, their modality of communication, quality of self-expression, object use and interactions, cause and effect, vocabulary, grammar, and phrase length.
- Pragmatic/Social Language assesses a student's use of communicative intent; questioning skills; conversational skills;

turn-taking; topic initiation, maintenance, and elaboration; appropriateness of communication; reading/literacy; writing/ spelling; and memory.

◆ Speech evaluates a student's overall speech intelligibility, oral motor structures, and their functions as they relate to speech sound production.

◆ Voice assesses the student's loudness, vocal quality, and pitch.

◆ Oral assesses the student's oral skills as they relate to daily functions such as mouth breathing, drooling, tongue thrust, and swallowing/ diet.

◆ Fluency assesses the student's fluency, rate of speech, and rhythm and intonation.

◆ Non-Oral Communication examines the student's use of sign language, two-dimensional expression, yes/no, fine-motor abilities, and effectiveness of current augmentative or alternative communication system.

Identification of Communicative Functions and Means. Children who are nonverbal often communicate in many other ways. For students who are non-verbal or have limited communication skills as a part of the evaluation process it is important to take an inventory of how (Communicative Means) and why (Communicative Functions) they communicate. Communicative functions or reasons for communicating may be expressed using a wide range of communicative means or ways to communicate including actions and behaviors. The following will provide a brief discussion, including specific examples, of both of these important aspects of communication.

Communicative Means. Communicative Means (ways to communicate) can be categorized as preverbal and verbal. Verbal means of communication include immediate echolalia, in which the child immediately repeats what was just spoken, and delayed echolalia, in which the child repeats what was heard earlier in the day or on a previous day. The use of single words and multiword utterances are examples of more advanced forms of verbal communication. Table 3–3 provides a brief description of the various preverbal means of communication a child may exhibit.

Communicative Functions. Of greater importance relative to communication are the purposes for which young children communicate. The communication attempts of early communicators generally serve three basic functions: *behavior regulation, social interaction*, and *joint attention* (Wetherby & Prizant, 1989). Young children exhibit "behavior regulation" when their communicative acts serve to regulate the behaviors of others. Behaviors and actions used to interact socially with another person, such as gaining someone's attention, are examples of social interaction types of communicative acts. Examples of communicative behavior used to establish joint attention include those used to direct another's attention or share information (Table 3–4).

Table 3–3. Preverbal and Nonverbal Means of Communication

Means of Communication	Description/Example
Physical Manipulation	Touches an object or toy repeatedly in an attempt to operate or activate
Giving	Gives an item to another person for a specific purpose (e.g., request assistance with activating a toy or open a closed container, or express an interest in the item)
Pointing	The child points to an item. This may serve a variety of communicative purposes, including to request or direct attention.
Showing	Shows an item but not for the objective of "giving" it away
Gaze Shift	Looks briefly in the direction of an item out of awareness
Proximity	Moves nearer or farther away from an item out of interest, or to get away from or protest
Head Nod/Head Shake	Indicates interest in or approval of an object by nodding, or protesting by shaking head
Facial Expression	Expresses emotion through facial expressions (e.g., smiling, frowning)
Self-Injury	Engages in self-injurious behaviors (e.g., hitting, biting, and banging) frequently in protest or to express the need to withdraw from an activity or situation
Aggression	Exhibits aggressive behaviors directed toward others (e.g., hitting, biting, punching, kicking, and scratching)
Tantrum	Screams and/or, throws self-down on floor usually to protest.
Crying/Whining	Cries and whines to express needs
Vocalizing	Expresses speech-like sounds that are not full words
Word Approximations	Attempts word approximations such as "wa-wa" for "water"

Source: Adapted from Wetherby (1995).

Table 3–4. Definitions of Communicative Functions and Application to Emergent AAC Users

Behavior Regulation

Category	Definitions	Discourse Structure	AAC Examples
Request Object	These are acts or utterances used to demand a desired tangible object. This includes requesting consumable and non-consumable items.	AAC user requests object and waits to receive desired object	I want XXX, want more, want that, yes (in response to question prompt—"Do you want?"), I need glue, more bubbles
Request Action	These are acts or utterances used to command another person to carry out an action. This includes requesting assistance and other actions involving another person or between another person and an object.	AAC user requests action and waits for response	Open, you push, you go, I go, read it, I need help, you do it, make go, more go, come here, again, do it again, turn, you turn
Protest	These are acts or utterances used to command another to cease an undesired action. This includes resisting another's action and rejection of object that is offered.	AAC user protests and waits for response	No, stop it, no go, no turn, no want, I don't like, no read

Social Interaction

Category	Definitions	Discourse Structure	AAC Examples
Greet	These are acts or utterances used to gain another's attention to indicate notice of their presence. These include greetings, calling, and conversational devices such as politeness markers and boundary markers.	AAC user makes a comment and may or may not wait for response	The child waves or says "Hi" when adult enters the room. The child shouts "Mom" when his or her mother is across the room to get her attention.

Greet *continued*		Non-AAC user makes a comment (or act) and AAC user follows up with an appropriate response	The child gives the adult a kiss or signs "Thank you" after the adult gives a desired object to the child waves "Bye" or uses symbols "I here"
Participation in Social Routine	These are acts or utterances used to command another to commence or continue carrying out a game or social interaction. These are acts or utterances used to participate in a game or social routine. This specific type of action request involves an interaction between another person and the AAC user, usually centered around a game or fun-oriented social interaction.	AAC user makes a request or comment and waits for response	Want chase, you do it, my turn, your turn, you go, I go
Showing Off	These are acts used to attract attention to something or something they are doing in an effort to say, "look at me."	AAC user addresses person (not object) and waits for response	Look here, I did it!
Request Permission	These are acts or utterances used to seek another's consent to carry out an action.	AAC user requests consent, waits for a response, and then responds by carrying out the action	I turn, I go potty, I do it, glue on?
Completion of a Verbal Script	These are acts or utterances used to complete a verbal script.	Non-AAC user provides a verbal script, leaving off the final word or phrase and AAC user completes the script	Ready, set GO, or 1, 2, THREE, Take it OFF

continues

49

Table 3–4. *continued*

Joint Attention

Category	Definitions	Discourse Structure	AAC Examples
Comment	These are acts or utterances used to direct another's attention to an object or event. These include showing, describing, informing, and interactive labeling.	AAC user makes a comment directed towards an object or event; may or may not wait for a response.	I like that, I don't like that, I feel bad/good, no like (commenting not protesting, sharing a preference), no (in response to do you like?")
Ask Question	These are utterances used to find out something about an object or event. These include wh-questions and other utterances having the intonation contour of an interrogative.	AAC user asks a question and waits for response	What that? Where go? Do you like play?
Respond to Question	These are acts or utterances in response to a question posed by another.	Non-AAC user asks a question and AAC user responds	Responds to "What is that?" "What's your name?" Does not include responding to question request (e.g., "Do you want cookie?") or prompt question to retell past event or share upcoming event
Share a Past or Future Experience	These are acts or utterances to retell a past experience or notify about an upcoming experience.	AAC makes comment and may or may not wait for response	I go movie, I eat that, I go lunch

Sources: Adapted from Wetherby & Prutting, 1984; Wetherby, Cain, Yonclas, & Walker, 1988.

Communication Matrix. The Communication Matrix is a free online assessment measure created to help families and professionals easily understand the communication status, progress, and unique needs of anyone functioning at the early stages of communication, or using forms of communication other than speaking (Rowland, 2016). Someone familiar with the child describes various communicative behaviors exhibited by the child (e.g., Unconventional Communication, Conventional Communication, Concrete Symbols, etc.) and the function of those behaviors (e.g., to refuse, to obtain something, for social purposes, and to gain information). Specific communicative behaviors and messages are identified as not used, emerging, or mastered. Upon completion of the survey, a one-page profile is generated illustrating the child's communication status at a glance, along with a "Communication Skills List" that shows the specific communicative behaviors the individual uses. The matrix gives both a qualitative description of the child's current communicative functioning, as well as a quantitative description of which developmental age range their communicative abilities fall within. This assessment tool is currently available in English, Spanish, Chinese, Russian, Korean, and Vietnamese (https://www.communicationmatrix.org/).

The Triple C: Checklist of Communication Competencies, Revised. There are very few assessment tools specifically developed to assess adolescents and adults who are functioning at the emergent level of communication. The Triple C: Checklist of Communication Competencies, Revised (Bloomberg, West, Johnson, & Iacono, 2009) is one such tool. It was designed to assess the communication skills of adolescents and adults with severe to multiple disabilities who are emergent communicators functioning at the pre-intentional non-symbolic level progressing to greater levels of intentional symbolic communication. The checklist, typically completed by those familiar with the individual, including classroom teachers and caretakers, examines communication at five stages: *unintentional passive communication*, *unintentional active communication*, *intentional informal communication*, *basic symbolic communication*, and *established symbolic communication*. At the unintentional passive stage, meaning is assigned to behaviors exhibited by an individual in response to either external or internal stimuli by those familiar to the individual. At the unintentional active stage, although communicative intent continues to be imposed on the individual's behaviors by those familiar to them, the emergent communicator is purposefully acting on objects. For example, given a choice of food items, the emergent communicator will be observed to reach for the preferred item of choice. At the intentional informal stage, the emergent communicator utilizes non-formal forms of communication, such as gestures, to fulfill wants and needs. At the basic symbolic and established symbolic stages of communication, the emergent communicator is expanding their use of conventionally recognized symbolic forms of communication.

The Triple C: Checklist of Communication Competencies Revised takes approximately 15 to 45 minutes to complete. Items are identified as observed or not observed. Upon completion of the checklist, ideas for developing communication skills through the various stages can be found in the manual InterAACtion: Strategies for Intentional and Unintentional Communicators (Bloomberg, West, & Johnson, 2004).

SCERTS Model. The SCERTS Model is a systematic and semi-structured, yet flexible, educational approach for children with autism spectrum disorders (Prizant, Wetherby, Rubin, Laurent, & Rydell, 2006). The SCERTS Assessment Process (SAP), which was developed as a component of the SCERTS Model to measure progress and meaningful change, is a criterion-referenced tool that directly links assessment to educational and intervention planning. This tool is particularly useful in gathering specific information in the areas of joint attention and communicative means with students whose skills are not easily measured using many standardized tests. The SCRETS Model considers communication based on a three-stage developmental continuum: Social Partner Stage, Language Partner Stage, and Communication Partner Stage. Children with CNNs who the intervention approach described in this book was developed for typically fall within the Social Partner and Language Partner Stages. Within each one of these stages, this curriculum-based assessment examines skills in three domains: Social Communication, Emotional Regulation, and Transactional Support. The Social Communication domain is divided into two core components: Joint Attention and Symbol Use. Parents, teachers, and therapists who interact with the child are involved in the assessment process by contributing to the information about the child's abilities, strengths, and weaknesses in naturalistic, everyday activities. All these witnesses provide important information about how the child responds to and initiates social interactions.

Symbol Use. Symbol Use as it relates to the SCERTS assessment process (SAP) is a component of the Social Communication domain of the SCERTS model, and encompasses a child's use of symbols, specifically how the child uses and understands the symbols of communication. Within the onset of the Social Partner Stage, skills related to the child's ability to learn through imitation, as well as early forms of communication are identified. At the Conversational Partner Stage, (the highest of the three stages of the developmental continuum) skills such as the ability to understand and use advance relational words (e.g., wh-question words and prepositions), along with the ability to understand and use complex sentence structures, are examined. Table 3–5 provides an overview of the skills in symbol use, which are examined at both the Social Partner and Language Partner Stages.

Joint Attention. The authors apply the term joint attention, a core deficit of many children who will benefit from the intervention approach described in this book, two different ways. First, they describe joint attention as, "a child's ability to engage in reciprocal interactions with a variety of partners" (Prizant et al., 2006, p. 21). Secondly, they relate joint attention to the child's ability to "bring another person's attention to an interesting object or event by

Table 3–5. Overview of Symbol Use at the Social Partner and Language Partner Stages of the SCERTS Assessment Process (SAP)

Social Partner Stage	Language Partner Stage
Learns by imitation of familiar actions and sounds	Learns by observation and imitation of familiar and unfamiliar actions and words
Understands nonverbal cues in familiar activities	Understands nonverbal cues in familiar and unfamiliar activities
Uses familiar objects conventionally in play	Uses familiar objects conventionally in play
Uses gestures and nonverbal means to share intentions	Uses gestures and nonverbal means to share intentions
Uses vocalizations to share intentions	Uses words and word combinations to express meaning
Understands a few familiar words	Understands a variety of words and word combinations without contextual cues

Source: Prizant, Wetherby, Rubin, Laurent, & Rydell, 2006

commenting, requesting information, or providing information" (p. 21). This last application of joint attention exemplifies one of the primary goals of the intervention approach described in this book, and that is to move emergent communicators toward greater levels of social competency as demonstrated by their ability to use their communication systems for purposes that extend beyond behavioral regulation forms of communication. Table 3–6 provides an overview of the skills in the area of joint attention that are examined at both the Social Partner and Language Partner Stages.

Communication Sampling and Analysis. Children with complex communication needs, such as those who are nonverbal, do in fact communicate; however, their means of communication are frequently unconventional and not easily recognized. The Communication Sampling and Analysis (CSA), (Buzolich, Russell, Lunger-Bergh, & Burns-McCloskey, 2011) is an online assessment tool designed for infants, toddlers, and children with multiple physical, sensory, speech, and cognitive/linguistic challenges. This objective measure allows a clinician to objectively sample and analyze, in naturalistic interactions, the communicative behaviors and the functions of behaviors demonstrated by nonverbal or severely speech-impaired children, often a difficult group to assess. The CSA tool samples the communication behavior of the child with a partner in context during interactive activities. Observable communication behaviors (nonverbal, vocal, verbal), and the consequences or effects of those behaviors on their communication partner, are sampled. An inventory of the child's communication skills is developed. A clinician can

Table 3–6. Overview of Joint Attention at the Social Partner and Language Partner Stages of the SCERTS Assessment Process (SAP)

Social Partner	Language Partner
Engages in reciprocal interaction	Engages in reciprocal interaction.
Shares attention	Shares attention
Shares emotion	Shares emotion
Shares intentions to regulate behavior of others	Shares intentions to regulate behavior of others
Shares intention for social interaction	Shares intention for social interaction
Shares intentions for joint attention	Shares intentions for joint attention
Persists and repairs communication breakdowns	Persists and repairs communication breakdowns
	Shares experiences in reciprocal interaction

Source: Prizant, Wetherby, Rubin, Laurent, & Rydell, 2006

then utilize the inventory to demonstrate a need for a communication system (unaided and aided), develop intervention goals and objectives, train partners, and engineer the environment to increase communication opportunities. The CSA is useful as both a pre- and post-intervention tool that can be used to document progress, and ultimately justify continued treatment. Additionally, the online analysis creates a printable report that can be included in an evaluation report. It is also possible for a clinician to compare the student's current assessment from previous assessments or samples.

Identify Communication Needs

The next step of the AAC assessment process is to identify the communication needs of the potential AAC user. This is accomplished by comparing an individual's current means of communication, which was discussed in the previous section, to the communication demands of the various environments and activities in which they are expected to participate. This is a critical step of the assessment process that will not only guide the team in selecting the appropriate AAC system, but will influence how the AAC user will be taught to use their communication system.

Communication Demands and Opportunities Inventory. Students with CCNs participate in numerous activities and tasks with a wide range of communication partners throughout their school day. Each event or activity presents with unique expectations and potential opportunities to communicate. In order to understand the breadth of these communication demands and opportunities, it is necessary to observe the student over the course of several activities; a full day is preferred. The Communication Demands and Opportunities Inventory (Dodd, 2017, refer to accompanying website) was developed to document, organize, and put these observations into action. This inventory serves dual functions related to assessment and intervention implementation. The data and information gleaned from observing the student engaged in various activities will be used to directly link assessment findings to intervention implementation. Given the completed inventory, specific communicative acts and necessary vocabulary will be outlined and ready for the intervention team to implement. To begin, select several activities to observe and list them in the "activity" column. As the student is observed engaging in these various activities, the observer records any communication attempts exhibited by the student and level of support (e.g., hand-over-hand, indirect prompt) necessary to execute them. Refer to Chapter 6 for a discussion on potential levels of support and prompts. Next the observer notes communication expectations of the events and activities and potential communication opportunities. The observer completes the inventory by listing core and fringe vocabulary required for the student to actively participate in the activity or event.

Social Networks Communication Inventory. Another tool to consider is Blackstone and Hunt Bergs (2012) Social Networks: Communication Inventory for Individuals with Complex Communication Needs and Their Communication Partners. This inventory is an assessment and intervention-planning tool developed to identify the unique communication demands of individuals with complex communication needs, and complements Beukelman and Mirenda's (2013) Participation Model of Assessment previously discussed in this chapter. The Social Networks Communication Inventory examines the environments and individuals with whom the AAC user will most likely be communicating with, and identifies the communication skills needed to be successful in these different situations. Using this inventory communication needs are considered within five categories or "circles." Circle 1 is the inner circle and includes parents and siblings. Circle 5, the outer circle, includes unfamiliar persons the student will encounter. An AAC user's social networks will change throughout their lives.

Social Networks Communication Inventory

Circle 1: Life Partners—parents and siblings

Circle 2: Friends and Relatives—grandparents, classmates

Circle 3: Acquaintances

Circle 4: Paid Workers—speech-language pathologist, teachers, occupational therapists

Circle 5: Unfamiliar Persons—doctors, dentists, restaurant staff

Assessment of AAC-Related Skills

The final aspect of the appraisal piece of the assessment process is to examine skills related to AAC use. Prior to recommending a particular AAC system, it is important to understand the student's proficiency in various AAC-related skills, such as the ability to select icons from a field of pictures, and to navigate between levels. Dynamic assessment (previously introduced in this chapter) is an important component of assessing AAC related skills. In application, present levels and abilities are identified and the student's likelihood to further develop or refine specific skills is considered when the assessment team makes specific recommendations related to an AAC system.

Each communication system—technology- and non-technology-based—is comprised of features that make it unique and customizable. Feature matching is a common technique used to "match" the ability and needs of the potential AAC user with the most appropriate AAC system, device, and/or techniques. Table 3–7 provides a list of features that are often considered when matching an AAC user's needs and abilities to an appropriate AAC system.

There are a number of criterion-referenced tasks and checklists to assess and identify various AAC-related skills. The following provides a discussion of some of those.

AAC Profile™: A Continuum of Learning. The AAC Profile (Kovach, 2009) is an ongoing assessment tool that can be used to establish baseline performances prior to the implementation of the intervention and as a means to monitor and document progress periodically. Assessment items are divided hierarchically into ability-based levels called Skill Set Levels in four areas of learning. The four areas of learning correspond to Light's (1989) areas of communicative competence. Skill Set Levels range from simple and early functioning to independent use and AAC-system mastery. Behaviors are identified as occurring frequently and independently, sometimes often needing assistance, or seldom, even with support. The following is a discussion of each area of learning.

Operational Area of Learning. This area of learning assesses the development of the technical skills used to operate the AAC system. Skill Set Levels include Orientation and Awareness, Manipulation, Focused Use, AAC System Navigation, and AAC System Programming and Use.

Linguistic Area of Learning. This area of learning assesses the development of receptive and expressive language skills used in the home and community, the knowledge and use of the language "code" of the AAC system, and the ability to attend to both during a communicative interaction. Skill Set Levels include Communication Awareness, Communication with Specific Meaning, Communication by Combining Words, Communication Using Syntax and Morphology, and Communication Using Refined Language.

Table 3–7. Description of AAC Feature

AAC Feature	Description
Vocabulary Representation Method	This feature refers to the method or methods used to represent language in an AAC system. Single-meaning pictures, alphabet-based systems, and semantic compaction are the three basic methods used.
Symbol System	This feature refers to the type of symbols represented in an AAC device or system. These include unaided and aided symbols that range from low to high tech and can include real photos, or color or black and white drawings.
Output Modes	This feature refers to how information is sent out to communication partners. Synthesized speech (recorded human voice), digitized speech (computer-generated), and visual outputs (picture icons) are the most common modes.
Display	This feature refers to how symbols are displayed and/or organized and accessible to the AAC user. Fixed, dynamic, hybrid, and visual scene displays are the four most common display types.
Correctability of Message	This feature allows the AAC user to "clear" and/or "delete" entire sentences, individual words, or single letters as needed.
Construction and Durability	This feature refers to the ability of a device or display to withstand daily use and last for a long period of time, and withstand normal wear and tear.
Access/Selection Method	This feature refers to how the AAC user will control their device and select items for communication.
Future Expansion Capabilities	This feature allows users to delete or expand features and vocabulary in order to accommodate their present and future communication needs.
Word Predictability	This feature refers to a process that tries to guess the word a user is writing at the same time he/she is doing it. It is used to enhance the user's communication efficiently.

Source: Adapted from Beukelman & Mirenda, 2013.

Social Area of Learning. This area of learning assesses the development of skills needed for social communication, including the individual's self-image as a communicator, and the desire to communicate reciprocally with others. Skill Set Levels include Natural Behaviors, Effective Regulatory Behaviors, Practiced Interaction, Social Awareness and Competence, and Social Mastery.

Strategic Area of Learning. This area of learning assesses the knowledge of what can be communicated and how best to communicate it, as well as developing compensatory strategies for effective communication to account for the limitations imposed by the AAC system itself. Skill Set Levels include Pre-Intentional/Reflexive, Intentional, Programmed Message Use, Appropriate Message Selection and Use, and Strategic Mastery.

Test of Aided Communication Symbol Performance. The Test of Aided Communication Symbol Performance (TASP) (Bruno, 2010) is a non-standardized augmentative and alternative communication (AAC) assessment battery designed for individuals with complex communication needs. This test provides a starting point for designing or selecting an appropriate page set for an AAC device, designing communication boards, and determining appropriate intervention targets. Results are determined as percentages, based on the number correct out of the total, on the following subtests:

- Symbol Size and Number Subtest: This subtest determines the maximum number of symbols appropriate for a student to select from a display.
- Grammatical Encoding Subtest: This subtest determines what the student knows and understands. Action verbs (sleep, eat, wash), opaque verbs (e.g., get, make), people or actors, adjectives and adverbs (dry, hot, mad), prepositions, pronouns, locations, and articles are tested.
- Categorization Subtest: This subtest determines how the student can classify words into categories, which is useful for organizing topical and sub-topical page selection sets. Categorization skills are determined based on categorization tasks; basic superordinate categories, visualization categorization, auditory categorization, and category closure sentences.
- Syntactic Performance Subtest: This final subtest examines the student's ability to combine and sequence symbols to produce sentences. It tests a variety of sentence structures including simple two-word utterances, "Boy wash," three and four-word sentences, and present progressive sentences such as, "The girl is washing the doll." Use of articles and prepositions are also sampled. These sentences are based on a series of photographs, and the student is instructed to point to the corresponding photographs verbally presented by the examiner in sentence and question form (e.g., "Point to 'girl-play'"; "What does the baby do when he is hungry?") This subtest also includes a picture description task in which the client is asked to make up a sentence describing a photo.

AAC Evaluation Genie. The AAC Evaluation Genie is an informal assessment iPad app that is used for identifying skill areas related to the language

Table 3–8. *AAC Evaluation Genie:* Description of Subtests

Subtest	Description
Visual Identification	Evaluates a student's ability to visually track and identify a single icon from 5 inches and a field of 2 items to 1 inch in size and a field of 32 items
Visual Discrimination	Evaluates a student's ability to visually track and discriminate a single icon from a field of two five-inch items icons to a field of 32 one-inch items
Noun Vocabulary	Evaluates a student's ability to identify common noun vocabulary
Function Vocabulary	Evaluates a student's ability to identify common noun vocabulary stated by function
Verb Vocabulary	Evaluates a student's ability to identify common action word vocabulary
Category Recognition	Evaluates a student's ability to identify common noun vocabulary by category group inclusion
Word Association	Evaluates a student's ability to identify a noun by associated feature of function
Category Inclusion	Evaluates a student's ability to identify common noun vocabulary by category inclusion
Picture Description	Evaluates a student's ability to describe basic pictures using a simulated AAC display

Source: Helling, 2016

representation methods commonly found on AAC systems. This assessment consists of 14 subtests in the domains of visual skills, vocabulary skills, and core vocabulary knowledge. Table 3–8 provides description of each subtest and the skills assessed in each.

Interpret Assessment Findings and Make Recommendations

The final step of the assessment process, as it relates to AAC, is to translate the data and information gathered during the appraisal phrase into recommendations specific to both the AAC system and intervention implementation. At the end of the assessment process, it is important to make a clear recommendation related to the type of AAC system and/or strategies that will best meet the needs of the student. Chapter 4 continues the discussion of selecting the most appropriate AAC system. Depending on the type of AAC system recommended, it may be necessary to make specific recommendations regarding how the AAC system will be programmed to facilitate its use. Refer to the Chapter 4 discussion on "Principles of Programming to Support Acquisition of Communication" to develop this section of your recommendations. It is important to make a clear recommendation regarding the training of all participants, including parents, teachers, and instructional support staff. Training sessions will need to be customized based on participants' educational and professional background, and the roles and responsibilities that will be assigned to them. Appendix A provides a list of training topics to consider when developing a training agenda. Goals in each competency area should be identified and developed. Refer to Chapter 6 for specifics in developing goals in each competency area. Conclude the recommendation with specific intervention techniques and strategies. These will be covered in detail in Chapter 5. Frequently, in the end it will be necessary to increase communication opportunities and language models. Both of these are discussed in detail in Chapters 4 and 5.

REFERENCES

American Speech-Language Hearing Association (ASHA). (2004). *Roles and responsibilities of speech-language pathologists with respect to augmentative and alternative communication* [Technical report]. Retrieved from http://www.asha.org/policy/TR2004-00262/

American Speech-Language Hearing Association (ASHA). (2016). *Assessment tools, techniques, and data sources*. Retrieved from http://www.asha.org/Practice-Portal/Clinical-Topics/Late-Language-Emergence/Assessment-Tools-Techniques-and-Data-Sources/

Beukelman, D. R., & Mirenda, P. (2013). *Augmentative and alternative communication: Supporting children and adults with complex communication needs* (4th ed.). Baltimore, MD: Paul H. Brookes.

Blackstone, S., & Hunt Berg, M. (2012). *Social networks: A communication inventory for individuals with complex communication needs and their communication partners, revised version*. Verona, WI: Attainment.

Bloomberg, K., West, D., & Johnson, H. (2004). *InterAACtion: strategies for intentional and unintentional communicators*. Australia: Box Hill.

Bloomberg, K., West, D., Johnson, H., & Iacono, T. (2009). *Triple C manual and checklists, revised*. Australia: Box Hill.

Bruno, J. (2010). *Test of Aided-Communication Symbol Performance*. Pittsburgh, PA: Dynavox Mayer Johnson.

Buzolich, M. J., Russell, D. B., Lunger-Bergh, J., & Burns-McCloskey, D. (2011) *Communication sampling and analysis*. Retrieved from http://csa.acts-at.com/

Carrow-Woolfolk, E. (2014). *Test of Auditory Comprehension of Language, 4th Edition (TACL-4)*. Austin, TX: Pro-Ed.

Darley, F. (1991). A philosophy of appraisal and diagnosis. In F. Darley & D. Spriestersbach (Eds.), *Diagnostic methods in speech pathology* (22nd ed., pp. 1–23). Prospect Heights, IL: Waveland Press.

Dodd, J. L. (2010). Thinking outside of the assessment box: Assessing social communicative functioning in students with ASD. *ASHA Division 16: Perspectives on School-Based Issues, 11*(3), 88–98.

Dodd, J. L., Franke, L. K., Grzesik, J. K., & Stoskopf, J. (2014). Comprehensive multidisciplinary assessment protocols for autism spectrum disorder. *Journal of Intellectual Disability: Diagnosis and Treatment, 2,* 68–82.

Fenson, L., Marchman, V. A., Thal, D. J., Dale, P. S., Reznick, J. S., & Bates, E. (2006). *MacArthur-Bates Communicative Development Inventories user's guide and technical manual* (2nd ed.). Baltimore, MD: Paul H. Brookes.

Helling, C. (2016). AAC Evaluation Genie (Version 2.7) [Mobile application software]. Retrieved from http://itunes.apple.com

Individuals with Disabilities Education Act, 20 U.S.C. § 1400. (2004).

Johnston, S. S., Reichle, J., Feelely, K. M., & Jones, E. A. (2012). *AAC strategies for individuals with moderate to severe disabilities.* Baltimore, MD: Paul H. Brookes.

Kleiman, L. (2003). *Functional Communication Profile. Revised.* East Moline, IL: LinguiSystems.

Kovach, T. M. (2009). *AAC Profile: A continuum of learning.* East Moline, IL: LinguiSystems.

Light, J. (1989). Toward a definition of communicative competence for individuals using augmentative and alternative communication systems. *Augmentative and Alternative Communication, 5*(2), 137–144.

Moore, B. J., & Montgomery, J. K. (2017). *Speech language pathologists in public schools: Making a difference for America's children* (3rd ed.). Austin, TX: Pro-Ed.

No Child Left Behind Act, 20 U.S.C. § 6319. (2001).

Popham, J. W., (1975). *Educational evaluation.* Englewood Cliffs, NJ: Prentice-Hall.

Prizant, B. M., Wetherby, A. M., Rubin, E., Laurent, A. C., & Rydell, P. J. (2006). *The SCERTS Model: A comprehensive educational approach for children with autism spectrum disorders.* Baltimore, MD: Brookes.

Quill, K. A. (2000). *DO-WATCH-LISTEN-SAY. Social communication intervention for children with autism.* Baltimore, MD: Brookes.

Quill, K. A., Bracken, K. N., & & Fair, M. E. (2000). *Assessment of Social Communication Skills.* Baltimore, MD: Brookes.

Rossetti, L. (2006). *Rossetti Infant-Toddler Language Scale.* Austin, TX: Pro-Ed.

Rowland, C. (2016). *The communication matrix.* Retrieved from https://www.communicationmatrix.org/

U.S. Department of Education. (2015). *Every Student Succeeds Act (ESSA).* Retrieved from http://www.2.ed.gov/policy/elsec/leg/essa/index.html

Every Student Succeeds Act S.117-114th Congress. (2015).

Westby, C. E. (2000). A scale for assessing development of children's play. In K. Gitline-Weiner, A. Sandgrund, & C. Schaefer (Eds.), *Play diagnosis and assessment* (pp. 15–57). New York, NY: John Wiley & Sons.

Wetherby, A., & Prizant, B. (2002). *Communication and Symbolic Behavior Scales Developmental Profile (CSBS:DP).* Baltimore, MD: Brookes.

Wetherby, A. M. (2003). *Communication and Symbolic Behavior Scales.* Baltimore, MD: Brookes.

Wetherby, A. M., Cain, D. H., Yonclas, D. G., & Walker, V. G. (1988). Analysis of intentional communication of normal children from the prelinguistic to the multiword stage. *Journal of Speech and Hearing Research, 31,* 240–252.

Wetherby, A. M., & Prizant, B. M. (1989). The expression of communicative intent: Assessment guidelines. *Seminars in Speech and Language, 10* (1), 77–91.

Wetherby, A. M., & Prutting, C. (1984). Profiles of communicative and cognitive-social abilities in autistic children. *Journal of Speech and Hearing Research, 27,* 364–377.

Zimmerman, I. L., Steiner, V. G., & Pond, R. E. (2011). *Preschool Language Scales* (5th ed.). San Antonio, TX: Pearson.

CHAPTER 4

Intervention Planning Phase

Prior to implementing an AAC-based intervention careful consideration is given to not only selecting and programming/developing the appropriate AAC system but allocating time allocated to engineering the environment and training facilitating participants so that an intensive, immersive, language-rich atmosphere is created. This chapter outlines what needs to occur during the intervention-planning phase to ensure effective implementation of the AAC intervention. Skipping this mediatory step—planning for the implementation of the intervention—could potentially jeopardize the student's ability to reach his or her potential.

During the intervention planning phase, critical decisions are made, not only regarding which AAC system is best suited to meet the communication needs of the student, but more importantly how the system will be developed, organized, and/or programmed. Careful consideration is given to the types of vocabulary that will be accessible to the student and how that vocabulary will be represented (e.g., visually) and organized. The environment is engineered to optimize the student's learning opportunities. Key professionals, referred to as communication guides, are trained in the fundamentals of AAC and related intervention practices. Lessons plans are carefully created to systematically teach key AAC skills. The intervention planning phase provides an opportunity to:

- ◆ Identify communication needs, taking into consideration information gleaned during the assessment phase or baseline measures
- ◆ Establish goals and desired outcomes based on communication needs
- ◆ Customize the student's communication system, taking into consideration their abilities (i.e., feature matching), needs, and intervention goals

- ◆ Engineer the environment to create a language-rich environment
- ◆ Prep for intervention implementation (e.g., training communication guides regarding intervention principles and implementation strategies, lesson planning)
- ◆ Prepare for generalization to occur

MOVING FROM ASSESSMENT TO INTERVENTION

Once all the data have been compiled during the assessment phase, the next step is to develop a plan for implementing the intervention program. Too often the "intervention planning phase" is bypassed without forethought as to how an AAC intervention program will be implemented. As a result, this can be one of the reasons the novice AAC communicator struggles to acquire the necessary skills to successfully and effectively use his or her AAC system. This includes not only selecting an appropriate AAC system, (technology- or non-technology-based), but will also include the time devoted to either programming or developing an AAC system that will meet the needs of the student and support their acquisition of communication.

Identification of Intervention Needs

The information gathered during the assessment phase is used to match the communication needs of the potential AAC user with an AAC system that will support their acquisition of communication. Consider the example of Jerome, a 16-year-old male who presented with a diagnosis of autism spectrum disorder. Throughout his educational experience, Jerome had been exposed to a myriad of interventions including picture-based communication systems with varying success. In spite of years of intervention, Jerome continued to be identified as a non-symbolic, non-intentional communicator who relied on: (a) behaviors (e.g., self-injurious behaviors, rocking); (b) vocalizations; (c) gestures (e.g., pushing food items away to indicate he did not like or want what was placed in front of him and/or to indicate he wanted something else); and (d) a few words or phrases he could imitate with reduced intelligibility (e.g., "I want cracker") to indicate wants and needs, and protest. Following an AAC evaluation, it was determined that Jerome would benefit from a communication system that would:

1. Support his acquisition of communication through the development of communicative intent, linguistic understanding, and expressive communication.
2. Provide a language system that facilitates early forms of communication and one that is easily understood.
3. Provide him with a means to communicate basic wants and needs.

4. Expand as his communication skills develop.
5. Offer an efficient and effective means to communicate with his family, peers, teachers, and people in the community.
6. Provide access to a variety of pragmatic language functions such as requesting actions and objects, commenting, directing others, signaling for help, greeting, protesting, asking questions, and sharing information with communication partners.

Moving forward with this information, the intervention team determined that Jerome would benefit from a speech-generating device that would give him access to a core vocabulary with activity-specific fringe words, including real photos of preferred objects and food items. Jerome's AAC system, a 5 × 5 dynamic grid display, included fringe words located in folders associated with "eat" and "favorite things." Jerome was initially taught to use his AAC system to request preferred food items, comment about preferences (e.g., "like," "no like," "no want"), and direct the behavior of his communication partners (e.g., "I go," "my turn") in congruence with his linguistic competency goals. Once the communication needs were established, the team could begin developing a plan for the implementation of an evidence-based intervention.

Establishing Intervention Targets

Another step of the intervention process that bridges assessment to intervention is establishing goals and objectives. Identifying what it is you want the AAC user to accomplish in response to the intervention lays the foundation of the intervention plan. Goals and objectives, although necessary—not to mention a mandated under federal law—for evaluating and monitoring a student's response to an intervention, serve an even more functional purpose. In fact, we may want to shift our perspective on goal setting from a mandate under federal law, to an opportunity to identify what it is we want a particular student to accomplish in a designated period of time. As Brian Tracy (2007) author of the book *Eat That Frog*, reminds us, "Goals are the fuel in the furnace of achievement" (p. 13). If the goal is to progress a student to greater levels of communicative competence, then it is important to develop goals in each one of the four competency areas. This following section provides a brief overview of goal-setting relative to each competency area. A more detailed discussion of how to write goals in each competency area, and how to monitor progress is presented in Chapter 6, *Progress Monitoring*.

Linguistic Competence

In addition to referring to the receptive and expressive language skills of the AAC user's native language(s), linguistic competence also encompasses their knowledge of the linguistic code of their AAC system (e.g., picture symbols, line drawings, real photos, words) (Light, 1989; Light & McNaughton, 2014). Writing goals in the area of linguistic competency shares many similarities to goals written in the area of expressive language. Acquiring skills in the area of linguistic competence requires students to expand their symbolic knowledge (semantics) and the ability to compose messages of increasing length and complexity (syntax and morphology).

Operational Competence

Operational competence refers to skills related to the technical operation and execution of both aided and non-aided AAC systems (Light, 1989; 2003; Light & McNaughton, 2014). Unaided forms of communication require individuals to demonstrate specific degrees of body control or manual dexterity to execute communicative behaviors such as manual signs, gestures, eye blinking, and head nodding. Both technology- and non-technology-based systems may require the individual to use their index finger or a pointer to directly select desired icons. For those AAC users with significant physical impairments, demonstrating the ability to use partner-assisted scanning or scanning with dual switches may be skills that need to be developed. For those individuals using non-technology-aided forms of communication, such as a communication book or board, operational skills may involve opening their communication book and locating an activity-related vocabulary page within the context of the appropriate environment or activity. Individuals using dynamic display types of AAC systems will need to demonstrate the ability to navigate between pages, along with other operational types of skills such as turning on/off their system, activating the message bar, and deleting the previous message. As the AAC user develops skills related to operational competence, more advanced skills may be introduced, such as the ability to correct and erase messages, and return to the home page. To increase ownership of use, individuals who are learning to communicate with the support of an AAC system should be in the practice of independently transitioning their AAC system to various activities throughout their day and, when necessary, knowing where to store, locate, and retrieve it when appropriate.

Social Competence

This refers to the communicative purposes for which the AAC user uses their communication system, and includes communication acts to control their environment (e.g. requesting preferred objects or actions, protesting), along with social interactive purposes (e.g., commenting, requesting information) (Wetherby & Prutting, 1984). Students with complex communication needs (CCNs) are routinely taught to communicate for purposes of requesting preferred objects or desired food items, but the challenge is expanding the use of their communication systems for more social communicative purposes. In addition to increasing the novice AAC user's responsiveness to bids for communication, it is important to increase their overall rate of initiation. Unfortunately, research has shown that individuals who use AAC tend to assume the role of responder with fewer opportunities to initiate communicative acts independently, (Beukelman & Mirenda, 2013). For the population of AAC users who are the target of the intervention approach described in this book, increasing these opportunities is even more imperative.

Strategic Competence

Strategic competence encompasses those skills the AAC user employs to compensate for the shortcomings of their AAC system. There are inherent limitations with any AAC system, and the AAC user must adapt to these. With an AAC system, communication attempts can be easily missed; therefore, it is necessary the novice AAC user implements strategies that will ensure their messages are received and/or understood. Demonstrating persistence until a desired outcome is obtained, modifying a communication signal that was either not received, was misinterpreted, or was unclear, along with waiting for a communication partner to respond to a communicative attempt, are all challenges exhibited in this subgroup of students with CCNs. AAC users who are described as "aloof" or "passive" in their communicative acts (Wing & Gould, 1979) will require direct instruction in recognizing when there is a failed communication attempt and how they can adapt or modify their approach to ensure their message is successfully received.

Mismatch Between Communication Goals and Opportunities

An inherent downfall of many well intended AAC-based interventions is the mismatch between goals and learning opportunities. At times, well-written goals and objectives are formulated without careful consideration of how these goals will be addressed throughout the student's day. The challenge is that what we want students to accomplish is not always supported by meaningful learning opportunities dispersed throughout their day. Consider the goal of a student expressing "all done" upon completion of an activity or goal. This goal is frequently written into individualized education programs (IEPs) for students who use picture symbols to communicate. The question arises, "How often does the student have the opportunity to observe the symbol 'all done' (used to indicate completion) in the context of their daily routine?" The answer is probably not very often, if at all. Frequently, facilitating adults will use the manual sign for "all done" at the end of a story, circle time, or snack time, but rarely use the picture symbol of "all done." One way to incorporate "all done" is to attach the picture symbol for "all done" at the end of books. Another opportunity is to include "all done" on the student's visual schedule, which is discussed in more detail later in this chapter. As previously discussed in this book, students must experience their language system multiple times before they can ever be expected to use it.

DEVELOPING AN AAC SYSTEM TO SUPPORT ACQUISITION OF COMMUNICATION

In order to facilitate a student's progression toward communicative competence, it is necessary to devise or configure an AAC system that will support their movement forward toward increased levels of communicative competence. This begins with selecting the appropriate AAC system, whether a non-technology- or technology-based system. Each AAC user presents with a unique set of abilities and needs, and not all AAC systems will meet the needs of all AAC users equally. Therefore, careful consideration must be given to the AAC user's communication needs and abilities. Once a decision has been made regarding the specific AAC system, then time must be dedicated to how the AAC system is developed or programmed so that it aligns with the student's goals.

Selecting an Appropriate AAC System

With the advancement of technologies, the available AAC options have expanded exponentially. AAC teams, however, must proceed methodically in selecting the appropriate AAC system that matches the skills of the user and their communication needs. As introduced in Chapter 3, the selection process begins with a capability assessment. To review, a capability assessment refers to the process in which information is gathered related the AAC user's abilities in the areas of motor control, cognition, and literacy (Beukelman & Mirenda, 2013; Yorkston & Karlan, 1986). Aligning the student's needs and abilities to the different features of an AAC system through a process referred to as *feature matching* allows the team to systematically consider a range of AAC options, and ultimately, identify an AAC system that will best meet their needs.

At times, members of intervention teams may not agree as to what is the most appropriate AAC system for the individual. It is helpful to use a feature-matching chart (Table 4–1), to assist the team in coming to a consensus regarding which system best meets the student's needs. The chart lists the different AAC features, including a brief description of each feature and how the user's abilities and needs are related to the different specifications. The following is an example of how this information may be presented.

EXAMPLE: AAC Feature-Vocabulary Representation

Description. Vocabulary representation refers to the method or methods used to represent language in an AAC system. There are three basic methods used to represent language in an AAC system: single-meaning pictures, alphabet-based systems, and semantic compaction.

***Related to* Vocabulary Representation.** Carrie, a pre-symbolic communicator whose intentional communication is emerging, uses a gross approximated manual sign for "more," which she will produce as /mʌ/ in times of distress or in response to a communication partner's comments. With regard to her AAC system, Carrie needs access to single-word messages consisting of core vocabulary and activity-related fringe vocabulary.

The remainder of the chart outlines the various features of two to four AAC systems being considered as potential options for the AAC user. Displaying information in this manner gives the intervention team an objective perspective in considering their AAC options. In instances where team members have differing opinions of which AAC system is best suited to meet the needs of the student, the author has found it helpful to have each team member put an asterisk next to the three features they feel are most important, and then determine which AAC system appears to best meet the AAC user's needs with respect to those features. The author has found it beneficial to have the final decision be the team's decision. If everyone is in agreement, then the process of implementing the AAC system moves forward in a positive direction right from the beginning.

The Importance of Vocabulary Selection

Vocabulary plays a significant role in the way the AAC user utilizes his or her communication system. An AAC user who has a communication system comprised of pictures and icons of their favorite objects, food items, and activities will use their system for the purposes of requesting these items and activities. However, if the goal is for an individual to comment for the purposes of expressing preferences and dislikes and to share experiences, it is important that he or she have access to vocabulary that will afford them these kinds of communicative exchanges. This will provide them with the means to create phrases, such as "I like it" and "I don't like it." Equally, if a student's participation in age-appropriate games and activities is a target, then they will need to have the ability to create phrases such as, "My turn," Your turn," and "Do you have?" Therefore, the student will need to have access to vocabulary such as "turn," "my," "your," and "have."

Too often, the limited supply of symbols available to the student may deter their progress. Intervention teams often strive to expand the purposes for which the emergent AAC user utilizes their communication system, but fail to give them access to the necessary vocabulary for this to be accomplished. Therefore, it is critical a student have access to vocabulary that will enable them to use their communication system for an expanding range of communicative functions. Consider the communication board in Figure 4–1.

Table 4–1. Case Study: Carrie's Feature Matching Chart

AAC Features	Description of AAC Feature	Carrie's Abilities and Needs
Vocabulary Representation Method	This feature refers to the method or methods used to represent language in an AAC system. Single-meaning pictures, alphabet-based systems, and semantic compaction are the three basic methods used.	Carrie is a pre-symbolic communicator whose intentional communication is emerging. She uses a gross approximated manual sign for "more" and she will produce /mʌ/ in times of distress or in response to a communication partner's comments. Carrie needs access to single word messages consisting of core vocabulary and activity-related fringe vocabulary
Symbol System	This feature refers to the type of symbols represented in an AAC device or system. These include unaided and aided symbols that range from low to high tech.	Carrie is currently in a self-contained special day class. She has 1:1 instructional support throughout her day. She needs a symbol system (e.g., PCS) that can be supported throughout her day.
Output modes	This feature shows how information is sent out to communication partners. Synthesized speech (recorded human voice), digitized speech (computer-generated), and visual outputs are the most common modes.	Carrie is non-verbal. Carrie needs a speech-generating device that is easily recognizable and appealing to peers and familiar adults.
Display	This feature shows how symbols are displayed and/or organized and accessible to the AAC user. Fixed, dynamic, hybrid and visual scene displays are the four most common display types.	Carrie has not yet learned to navigate folders. Carrie needs a communication device with static display.

AAC Options

iPad with Proloquo2Go	iPad with TapSpeak	TouchChat	Go Talk 20+
Core vocabulary system (Word Spaces); includes categories, single-meaning pictures, automatic conjugation of verbs, plurals, and possessives for nouns, customization options	Single-meaning pictures arranged as single words and/or phrases	The VocabPC is arranged as carrier phrases, interactive sentences, activity vocabulary, and naming words. MultiChat15 uses sentences, phrases, individual words, interactive play, reading pages, and social pages. WordPower (word-based vocabulary).	Single-meaning pictures
SymbolStix, text-based	PCS, real photos, drawings	SymbolStix symbols, spelling, import photos and images	PCS, real photos, clip art
Synthesized	Digitized and synthesized speech; 20 languages and 43 voices. Auditory prompt (scanning) support. Separate voice/recording, speaking rate, and volume	Synthesized and digitized speech; 5 English synthesized voices	Digitized speech; volume control
Static or Dynamic	Static or Dynamic	Static or Dynamic	Static

continues

Table 4–1. *continued*

AAC Features	Description of AAC Feature	Carrie's Abilities and Needs
Correctability of Message	This feature allows the AAC user to "clear" and/or "delete" entire sentences, individual words or single letters as needed.	As an emergent communicator, Carrie will need to learn to be persistent (e.g., repeating her messages, gaining her communication partner's attention). Depending on the communication system she may need to learn to clear entire messages.
Construction and Durability	This feature refers to the ability of a device or display to last for a long period of time and withstand normal wear and tear.	Carrie is ambulatory and independent for mobility. She exhibits decreased muscle tone and coordination. She needs a device that is lightweight and easily carried (e.g., handle). Because of her motor weaknesses/sensory challenges, she needs a device that can withstand being dropped.
Access/Selection Method	The ways in which users control a device and select items for communication	Given a field of two, Carrie uses several fingers to indicate her preference. She has been learning to use an isolated index finger to select. Carrie frequently taps several times or maintains contact with a picture icon when selecting. Carrie needs a device that can be fitted with a key guard grid to increase fine motor accuracy.

	AAC Options		
iPad with Proloquo2Go	**iPad with TapSpeak**	**TouchChat**	**Go Talk 20+**
Delete/clear buttons	Backspace and clear message buttons; Double-tap message window to clear	Delete/clear buttons	None
This should be portable. Can be used on an iPhone, iPod Touch, and iPad. iMainGoX Case with an Integrated Speaker (featuring rechargeable lithium-ion battery), carrying strap, and USB power adapter for iPod Touch are available.	Static board grid dimensions (18 grid sizes to choose from). Dynamic grid resizing for quick board/page creation. Portable. Used on iPhone, iTouch, iPad	This should be portable. Protective cases available. Not as durable as other AAC devices. No warranty.	This should be portable and durable. Built-in overlay storage, Built-in handle,
Direct selection	Direct selection; one and two-switch scanning; single-message switch (tap response can be arranged to accommodate kids with varying motor skill levels). Touch/ Tap configuration: adjust the screen response to allow for a variable finger dwell on the surface	Direct selection; 12 location page layout	Direct Selection, Grids

continues

Table 4–1. *continued*

AAC Features	Description of AAC Feature	Carrie's Abilities and Needs
Future Expansion Capabilities	This feature allows users to delete or expand features and vocabulary in order to accommodate their present and future communication needs.	Carrie currently does not have a functional form of communication. She needs a communication system that will give her access to an increasing number of core vocabulary and activity-related fringe vocabulary.
Word Predictability	A process that tries to guess the word a user is writing at the same time he/she is doing it. It is used to enhance the user's communication ability.	This is not a feature that Carrie currently needs.

AAC Options

iPad with Proloquo2Go	iPad with TapSpeak	TouchChat	Go Talk 20+
Full expandability with 8000 symbols; customization options: item size, color, interactivity, restrictions, speech	There are up to 56 buttons on a board. Sequential-message switch for recording and playback of songs, stories, nursery rhymes, and other messages. Unlimited number of messages, sequence length, and phrase recording length. Create folders for each student or for various situations.	Customizable vocabulary, personalized pages, iShare subscription to share page sets	Has the ability to move, resize, rotate, and crop images to fit. Ability to change the text color, size and style. 45 message capacity. Uses AA batteries.
Multiword prediction	None	Word prediction	None

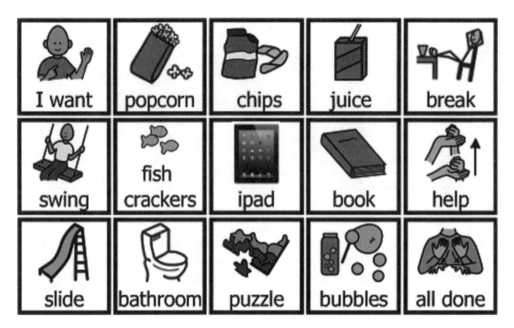

Figure 4–1. Communication Board: Fringe Vocabulary Words. The Picture Communication Symbols ©1981–2015 by Mayer-Johnson LLC, a Tobii Dynavox company. All Rights Reserved Worldwide. Used with permission. Boardmaker® is a trademark of Mayer-Johnson LLC.

The following is a sampling of some of the sentence constructs that can be formulated when the student is given access to these symbols:

I want chips (fish crackers, book, puzzle . . .)	I want all done
I want more	I want break
More chips (fish crackers, juice . . .)	I want bathroom
I want help	

This communication board (Figure 4–1) provides the student with picture symbols to request preferred food items and objects, indicate completion of a task, and request assistance or a break. These behavior regulatory communicative acts enable the student to fulfill immediate wants and needs through directing the behavior of another person. Contrastively, consider the communication board in Figure 4–2.

The following is a sampling of some of the sentence constructions that can be formulated given this set of symbols

I want that	No help	I go (?)
Want more	I like that	You go

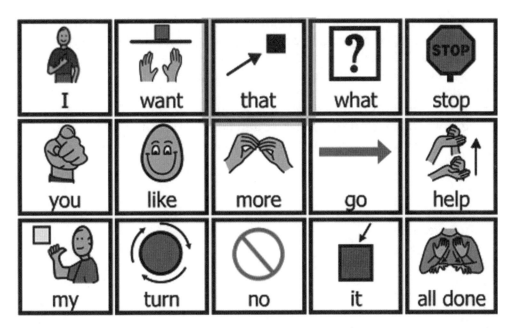

Figure 4–2. Communication Board: Core Vocabulary Words. The Picture Communication Symbols ©1981–2015 by Mayer-Johnson LLC, a Tobii Dynavox company. All Rights Reserved Worldwide. Used with permission. Boardmaker® is a trademark of Mayer-Johnson LLC.

No more	I no like that	My turn
I help	What that?	You turn it
I want help	No go	I turn in

A communication board (Figure 4–2) consisting of these words gives the student a means to request items and actions, express a preference, participate in a social routine, ask questions, and direct the behavior of another person.

The first communication board (see Figure 4–1) is composed predominately of fringe vocabulary words, and the second board (see Figure 4–2) is composed solely of core vocabulary words. Fringe vocabulary, sometimes referred to as content words (Hill & Romich, n.d.), are specific to activities and environments (Beukelman & Mirenda, 2014). For example, the terms crayons and scissors are specific to craft activities, whereas the terms stir and bowl are specific to cooking-related activities. Fringe words are individualized based on the communication needs of the individual. The following is a list of categories of fringe words that may be appropriate for a young child: common household objects (e.g., cup), preferred items, places (e.g., park), colors, body parts, and classroom materials.

Core vocabulary, on the other hand, refers to words that can be used across a variety of environments to convey an array of messages for a range of communicative functions (Beukelman & Mirenda, 2014). In fact, 85% of the words we use to communicate on a daily basis are composed of only a few hundred words (American Speech-Language-Hearing Association, n.d.). The earliest set of core vocabulary demonstrated in young children consists of pronouns (e.g., I), demonstratives (e.g., it, that), verbs (e.g., want), and prepositions (e.g., on, out) (Banajee, DiCarlo, & Buras-Sticklin, 2003). Surprisingly, fringe words that include object labels and nouns (e.g., car) are sparingly used by early communications. The following is a list of those words in order of prevalence.

1. I
2. No
3. Yes/yeah
4. Want
5. It
6. That
7. My
8. You
9. More
10. Mine
11. The
12. Is
13. On
14. In
15. Here
16. Out
17. Off
18. A
19. Go
20. What
21. Some
22. Help
23. All done/finished

As Beukelman, Jones, and Rowan (1989) determined, there is a preponderance of early communicators who use core vocabulary. As their study demonstrated, 25 of the most frequently occurring words used by preschoolers represented over 40% of the total different words used. Other core vocabulary words that are frequently exhibited in early communicators include *like, play, turn, eat, drink, happy, sad, come, do, make,* and *read*. Look for additional examples of core vocabulary in the examples provided throughout this chapter. Appendix B provides a list of core words frequently used by emergent communicators, including their definition(s) and application to AAC. For an expanded list of core vocabulary, including strategies to extend vocabulary to 300+ words refer to Van Tatenhoven (2005).

A unique feature of core vocabulary is its multifunction word use. Whereas fringe words typically serve a single function, many core vocabulary words possess multiple meanings. For example, the word "turn" can serve several functions depending on how it is used or which words it is paired with. A child may use the term "turn" to request an opportunity to turn the page of a book ("my turn") versus the physical action of turning the page ("I turn page"). Similarly, the word "like" can be used to request a turn ("I like turn"), to indicate a preference ("I like it"), and to describe similarities ("Do it like me").

Unfortunately, there is a tendency to avoid core words in the development of early communication boards and systems in part because they are generally difficult to represent in pictorial form. However, it is possible to teach children word-symbol association through modeling (e.g., aided language stimulation)—the picture meaning within the appropriate communication context. Knowing the importance core vocabulary plays on early communication attempts will assist intervention teams in developing a communication system that will support achievement of their goals.

Boards to Support Acquisition of Communication

Before discussing the specifics regarding setting up an AAC system, it is important to differentiate the different types of communication boards/pages that communication guides will utilize to facilitate the acquisition of their students' communication skills. The initial board or page is the *target board.* Target board refers to the communication board or home page that the team is ultimately striving to progress the emergent communicator to use. While it is difficult, if not impossible, to know exactly what the communication board or home page will look like following three or six months of intervention, however, it is important to have a preliminary target before you begin implementing intervention. As previously stated in this chapter, it is important to know your goal. Once the target board has been established a plan to progress the student toward the desired communication board or home page can be developed. This is important as we plan for intervention and ultimately begin strategically teaching the student to use their AAC system. This board will also serve the function of *modeling board.* A modeling board is a communication board the communication guide uses to model more advanced forms of language and language use. A student who is learning to communicate through the support of AAC system may initially be over whelmed by a communication system consisting of 25 picture icons (5 × 5 grid display) on a single page in spite of demonstrating the manual dexterity to access size cells typical of this type of grid display. In the initial stages of instruction, the student may only be able to manage two to four cells during any given activity. The downside is that the restricted number of symbols on this initial communication board/page limits the communication guide's ability to model more advanced language constructions. For example, during a gross motor activity involving "scooter boards, suppose the student has the following three symbols visible on their communication system: "want," "more," "no." However, the communication guide recognizes opportunities to model language such as "more go," "no more go," "I like," I don't like," but without access to these additional symbols (i.e., go, like, and don't) on the student's AAC system, the communication guide is limited in the number and types of language models they can model for the student. In summation, the student's communication system becomes a barrier to the communication guide's ability to model more complex language forms, or expand on the student's communication attempts. The symbols necessary to model more complex forms of language, or expand on the student's communication attempts, simply are not available. Having access to a communication board with a greater number of symbols gives the communication guide the symbols necessary to apply various language stimulation techniques such as modeling, expansionism, and self-talk (these are discussed in detail in Chapter 5, *Intervention Implementation*). The expanded modeling board also allows the communication guide to "talk" to the student using a parallel language to the one the student is learning to acquire.

In the initial stages of treatment, a student may find a communication board composed of 25 symbols or more overwhelming or distracting. This is particularly true for students who experience difficulty discriminating pictures. In these instances, the team may find the student benefits from simplified or condensed boards. Lesson boards, in many instances modified home pages, are ideal for focusing a student's attention to specific symbols that are the target of the current activity. The concept is the same regardless of the AAC system. For students whose AAC system is a non-technology-based communication system, it will be necessary to create separate lesson boards with only the target symbols showing. Many technology-based systems allow you to temporarily hide symbols that are not the focus of the current lesson. The important piece to remember is not to create a new communication board, but to modify the target/modeling board, ensuring the location of the icons is preserved. Consider the following communication boards. Figure 4–3 represents the target or modeling board whereas Figure 4–4 represents the icons available to the student during an activity involving scooter boards. In this instance, the student can use their abbreviated communication board to request go ("I go," "more go") and stop ("no more go"), express interest in the activity ("I like go," "I no like"), and instruct their communication guide to turn them around ("You turn it").

Creating Non-Technology-Based AAC Systems

Not all students will benefit from speech-generating devices; some students may do better with a non-technology-based AAC system, such as a communication board or book. Regardless, the same principles apply whether the communication system is technology-based or not. Begin with a base board consisting of primarily core vocabulary words and select fringe words (see

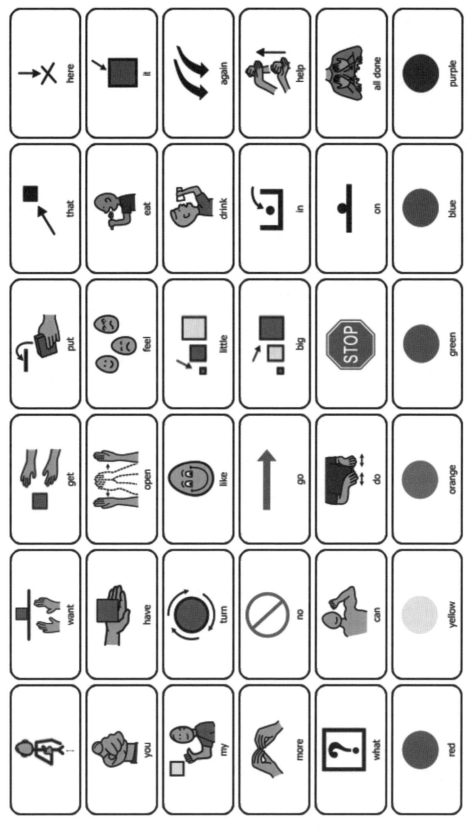

Figure 4–3. Target or Modeling Board. The Picture Communication Symbols ©1981–2015 by Mayer-Johnson LLC, a Tobii Dynavox company. All Rights Reserved Worldwide. Used with permission. Boardmaker® is a trademark of Mayer-Johnson LLC.

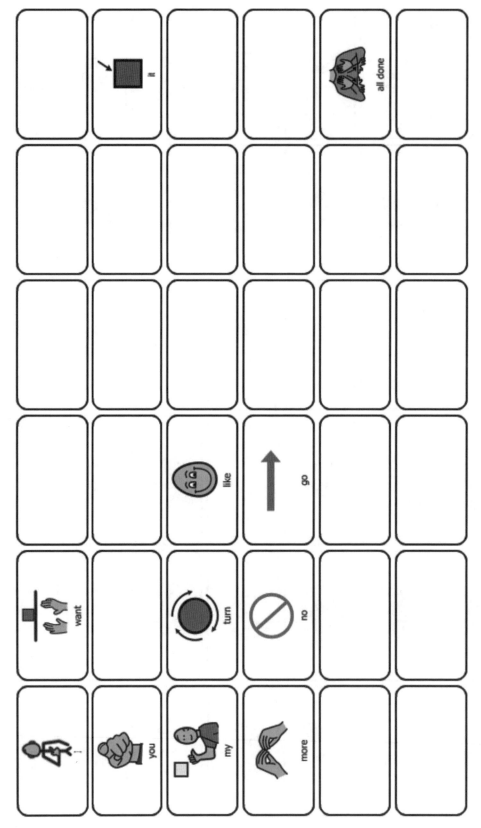

Figure 4–4. Lesson Board for Scooter Board Activity. The Picture Communication Symbols ©1981–2015 by Mayer-Johnson LLC, a Tobii Dynavox company. All Rights Reserved Worldwide. Used with permission. Boardmaker® is a trademark of Mayer-Johnson LLC.

Figure 4–3). It has been the author's experience that students in classroom-based settings often benefit from having access to colors and a symbol for bathroom, therefore these fringe words are frequently included on their base board. When creating the base board, it is important to leave a space at the top of the board so that strips of fringe words can be added and changed depending on the current activity or environment. The following is a list of potential school-related fringe strips:

Craft: Scissors, glue, paint, construction paper, crayons, paint, paint brush

Snack: Juice, water, crackers, fruit snack, cheese, banana, chips, fish crackers

Outside activities: Swing, slide, ball, monkey bars, chase

Story time: Book, page, read, listen, look, point

Feelings: Sad, happy, tired, mad, hungry, thirsty, bored

Communication Board

To create a communication board type AAC system, laminate the student's base board or adhere it to the back of a durable surface such as the back of a clipboard using packing tape or self-laminating sheets. You will want to leave a space at the top of the board for attaching fringe strips, using Velcro. This makes it easy to change vocabulary depending on the activity. A clipboard with a storage compartment works well for storing the fringe strips that will be changed depending on the activity.

Communication Flip Book

You can also create a flip book type communication book using a notebook binder, report folder, or having the pages spiral bound at your local print shop. To do this, begin with laminated copies of your core board and activity-specific fringe strips. When you create your core board leave, space at the top of your board for your fringe pages. Layer the fringe strips on top of the core board. This will give the student constant access to core words and the student can easily flip through the fringe strips depending on the activity. Color coding the fringe strips will give students quicker access to specific fringe strips as they learn to associate colors with specific activities.

Programming Technology-Based AAC Systems

Careful consideration must be given to how a device is programmed. Programming a student's device must align with their communication needs and desired intervention outcomes. Too often, the manner in which a student's AAC system is programmed is the crux to their success. There are two aspects with respect to programming that need to be independently considered: (1) technical aspects of programming, and (2) programming to support the acquisition of communication.

Technical Aspect of Programming a Communication System

The first facet of programming relates to the technical aspect of the AAC device or app. It is reasonable to expect that a multitude of individuals, who may include the speech-language pathologist, occupational therapist, classroom teacher, instructional staff, and parents, may at some point need to program the device; however, it is strongly encouraged that only a handful of individuals be assigned this responsibility. It has been the author's experience that if too many people are granted permission to program the student's AAC system, the organization or systematic programing of the device will eventually be compromised. Programming of the system must be intuitive and transparent. At any point, if someone on the intervention team strongly feels that a particular word should be added to the student's system, then sharing that with the appropriate person is encouraged so that it can be added in a logical manner. Although not everyone will be granted permission to program the system, it is important for everyone to understand how it is programmed. Understanding how a device or app is programmed gives better insight on how to use it and ultimately support the student's use of the communication system.

Each AAC device or app is uniquely different, however, there are features of programming which everyone should understand. In addition to knowing how to create and edit cells, it is important to understand how to create new pages and how to link pages. During instructional activities, knowing how to hide or temporarily delete cells will also be useful. Refer to the "AAC Technical Training Checklist" (Figure 4–5) for a list of the features that should be covered during the "Technical Aspect of Programming" training. This form can be used as a training checklist to ensure necessary features are covered during the training session.

Principles of Programming to Support Acquisition of Communication

The next facet of programming which will directly impact the student's acquisition of communication encompasses how picture icons are represented and organized on the AAC system itself. Continuing with the overarching goal of teaching the student to communicate with an AAC system, the following principles should be considered when programming or developing an AAC system.

Principle #1: Determine Number of Cells. Begin with determining the number of cells per page. This does not necessarily mean how many cells per

```
┌ ─ ─ ─ ─ ─ ─ ─ ─ ─ ─ ─ ─ ─ ─ ─ ─ ─ ┐
│                                   │
│        AAC Technical              │
│                                   │
│     Training Checklist            │
│                                   │
└ ─ ─ ─ ─ ─ ─ ─ ─ ─ ─ ─ ─ ─ ─ ─ ─ ─ ┘
```

Communication Guide	AAC Device/Program/App	Date of Training

AAC Feature	Complete	Notes
Create a new page or edit an existing page		
Select or change grid layout		
Change the number of cells per page		
Link cell to another page		
Link page back to home page		
Create or edit a cell		
Rearrange cells on a page		
Temporarily hide cell		
Delete a cell		
Edit picture icon label		
Change cell speech output		
Change cell actions		
Change cell activation timing		
Other:		
Other:		
Other:		
Other:		

AAC INTERVENTION: AN INTENSIVE, IMMERSIVE,
SOCIALLY BASED SERVICE DELIVERY MODEL

JANET L. DODD SLP.D., CCC-SLP
2016

Figure 4–5. AAC Technical Training Checklist.

page the student can currently manage, but more specifically the size of the cells. For example, if a student demonstrates the manual dexterity to access symbols on a 5 × 5 grid display, consider a 6 × 6 or 7 × 7 grid display, assuming with instruction, in a relatively brief period of time—for example three to four sessions—the student will develop the operational skills necessary to navigate through slightly smaller cells. The primary goal as it relates to number of cells is to begin with the maximum number of cells the student can currently manage or will learn to manage in a relatively short period of intervention. Having access to a larger set of symbols will initially give communication guides access to a larger number of picture icons for the purposes of modeling advanced forms of language and increasing language exposure opportunities.

Principle #2: Select Initial Set of Core and Fringe Words. Identify the student's initial vocabulary set. This should consist of primarily core vocabulary words and select fringe words. This initial word set should reflect the communication needs of the student and complement the communication opportunities encountered by them on a daily basis. This should have been, in part, identified during the assessment phase using various observation tools and interviews. For example, if one of the student's goals is to initiate using the restroom independently, then including a picture icon of "bathroom" would be appropriate. Although not a core vocabulary word, this particular picture icon is included based on the individual needs of the student. Table 4–2 provides a list of initial vocabulary words to consider; however, these are only guidelines or suggestions, taking into consideration an individual's motivation and functionality of words for that individual.

> Frequently, intervention teams want to ensure students have access to "yes" and "no." In order to make the most use of these words, we assume the student possesses the cognitive ability to understand and process "yes/no" question forms. However, for students who experience significant challenges understanding spoken language, the use of yes/ no is primarily limited to the purposes of indicating affirmation or rejection. For example, in response to questions such as "Do you want cookies?" or "Do you want to go outside?" a simple head nod or shake can suffice in response to these types of questions and is actually much more functional. If we apply the concept of "Prime Real Estate" (Principle # 8) we realize we do not want to take up valuable space on the student's core board with a word or symbol with limited application. However, it is important for the student to have access to negation ("no" or "not") because it can be used for a variety of communicative purposes, such as to cease an action ("no more" or "no go") or to indicate a preference ("I no like it").

Principle #3: Strive for Symbol Consistency. Individuals who use AAC rely on symbols rather than spoken words to communicate their needs, express their thoughts, and engage in conversation. Symbols represent words

Table 4–2. Core Vocabulary

Level 1 (10 words)	Level 2 (20 words)	Level 3 (30 words)	Level 4 (30+ words)
I	What	Put	More Action Words:
You	Turn	Get	
help	(My)	Open	Look
More	Here	Have	Put
Want	(Eat)	Can	Make
No/don't/not	(Drink)	Feel	Play
Stop	Do	In	Cut
That	Like	On	Colors
Go	It	Big	Additional Prepositions
Finished/ All done	Again	Little	Additional question words
		Good	
		Bad	He/She

to individuals who use AAC. Photographs, manual signs, colored pictures, black and white drawings, along with real objects are examples of some of the symbols frequently used by individuals who use AAC. Many of the students who are considered for this type of intervention model struggle with picture identification. Therefore, introducing the student to multiple symbol systems such as Boardmaker® and SymbolStix® shares the similar challenges as introducing an individual to multiple languages. To the maximum extent possible, use symbols for picture schedules and adapted stories consistent with the symbols on the student's communication system.

Principle #4: Select Universal Symbols. Since the goal is to teach the student the multifunction use of the different core vocabulary words, it is essential to select symbols with universal application. That is, they are not use-specific. The various symbol sets generally offer multiple options to choose from. For example, for the word "turn" Boardmaker® offers the options in Figure 4–6.

As Figure 4–6 demonstrates, Boardmaker® offers a wide selection of icons to represent the word "turn," some with very explicit application. For example, there are symbols to represent taking a turn in a game, a caterpillar turning into a butterfly, and turning a facet. Because the goal is for the student to use "turn" for all these different functions, it is important to select an icon with universal appeal. In this example, "c" would be the best choice.

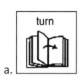 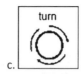 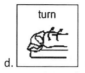 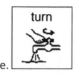 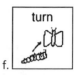

Figure 4–6. Various Uses of Turn. The Picture Communication Symbols ©1981–2015 by Mayer-Johnson LLC, a Tobii Dynavox company. All Rights Reserved Worldwide. Used with permission. Boardmaker® is a trademark of Mayer-Johnson LLC.

Principle #5: Represent Vocabulary as Individual Symbols. One of the purposes of introducing the AAC user to core vocabulary is to teach them the multifunction use of a word, which is characteristic of many core vocabulary words. In order to accomplish this, words must be represented as individual symbols. For example, "turn" can be combined with "my" to express "my turn" just as it can be combined with "on" to express "turn on." If "my turn" and "turn on" are represented in single picture icons as in the examples below (Figure 4–7), then the student is limited in the purposes for which they can use these symbols because of their narrow interpretation. Therefore, keeping in mind the goal of teaching multifunction word use of core vocabulary, it is essential the student have the ability to combine symbols with other symbols to create an expanding range of messages.

Principle #6: Strategically Place Symbols to Facilitate Language. To the maximum extent possible, place symbols in a manner that facilitates left-to-right message construction. This will not always work, as the functions of the words (e.g., from noun to verb) will change, depending on how they are used and/or how they are combined with other symbols.

> The Fitzgerald Color Coding Key was developed by Edith Fitzgerald in 1929, originally to teach hearing impaired individuals. The basic idea behind the key was a color coding classifying system for the different parts of speech. Since grammar is such an abstract concept, Edith Fitzgerald came up with the idea of adding color to classify different parts of grammar. This provided individuals with language difficulties a strategy to help them in identifying the different parts of speech. This does not work for the intervention approach described in this book, as many of the words assume varying grammatical functions, depending on how they are used.

Principle #7: Consistent Placement of Icons. Many students who are considered ideal candidates for the intervention described in this book experience significant difficulty not only with picture discrimination, but also the concept of symbol-to-object relationship. It is for this very reason that many of these stu-

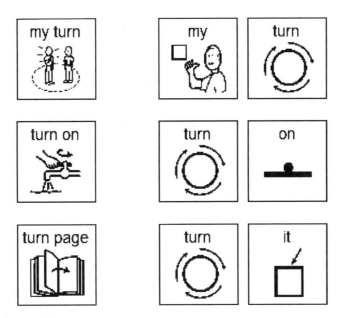

Figure 4–7. Single Versus Multiple Icons. The Picture Communication Symbols ©1981–2015 by Mayer-Johnson LLC, a Tobii Dynavox company. All Rights Reserved Worldwide. Used with permission. Boardmaker® is a trademark of Mayer-Johnson LLC.

dents are often not even considered candidates for AAC. But, as was discussed in Chapter 1, *Myths Dispelled*, these students learn object-symbol relationships through motor-planning instruction. Using a multisensory approach, students learn movement sequences to access vocabulary and construct messages. It is a very similar concept to the way one learns to type on a keyboard. Imagine one day if someone decided to move the keys around and you had to re-train yourself to a new configuration. To help our students, it is important we maintain a consistent placement of icons. It is for this reason that we want to strive for the maximum number of symbols (Principle #1) in the beginning. If it is decided to expand a student's communication system from a board or home page consisting of 25 symbols (5 × 5 grid), to one composed of 42 symbols (7 × 7 board), the original location of the symbol changes. For some students this would mean they would have to relearn the motor placements of the icons.

Principle #8: Apply Concept of "Prime Real Estate." The final principle to remember when programming or developing an AAC system for students with the most complex communication needs is the concept of "Prime Real Estate." For a multitude of reasons there are a group of students who struggle to expand their vocabulary or symbol knowledge. Therefore, we must ensure that each symbol on their AAC system serves a purpose. For this reason, it is important to periodically evaluate the student's symbol use to determine which symbols they are using the most often and which symbols they are only using sporadically or perhaps not at all. From there, determine if perhaps the reason they are not using a particular symbol is because they do not know how to use it or they are not given opportunities throughout their day to use it. If that is the case, then develop a plan to strategically teach the student how to use the particular symbol/word, and scaffold opportunities throughout the student's day so they can use it within real contexts. In the event it is determined that the symbol has very little value for this particular student, replace it with a word/symbol that will be of service to the student. Some students can only manage a restricted number of symbols; therefore, we want to ensure that each symbol on their communication system serves a purpose and is not simply occupying valuable real estate.

ENGINEERING THE ENVIRONMENT—VISUAL OPPORTUNITIES TO SEE SYMBOLS IN ACTION

Engineering the environment is one of the reasons this phase of the intervention process was included. Time needs to be set aside to create a language-rich environment so learning can occur. Students with CCNs have difficulty comprehending spoken language. It is not that they do not hear the words, but rather what they hear does not translate into a form of language they can comprehend. For some of these students. they are able to associate pictures and/or symbols to represent various forms of language. Furthermore, we recognize that "children learn to comprehend and produce words that are frequently spoken to them" (Harris & Reichle, 2004, p. 155), but how does that translate to children who are learning to communicate using a pictorial form? Students who are learning to communicate using an AAC system must experience language rich opportunities similar those experienced by children learning to communicate via spoken language. We do not always have to expect the student to communicate or use their communication systems all the time. They just need to be exposed to the language of their communication system. For this reason, it is important the student's environment be engineered to ensure these language exposure opportunities occur. The following are several examples of how to create a language-enriched environment, supportive of the language system the student is acquiring.

Modeling Board

Modeling boards, which were initially introduced earlier in this chapter, are expanded versions of the student's current communication system. They can be used by communication guides to model more advanced language forms and language use. Modeling boards provide a venue for the communication guide to employ various language stimulation techniques, such as self-talk and parallel talk using aided language modeling techniques. How to use modeling boards is discussed in detail in Chapter 5.

Visual Schedules

There is clear research evidence regarding the benefits of using visual schedules with individuals with autism spectrum disorders (ASD) (Bryan & Gast, 2000; Mesibov, Browder, & Kirkland, 2002), and other disabilities. Visual schedules capitalize on the visual strengths of these students using picture symbols as a receptive communication system to increase their understanding. An additional benefit of visual schedules specific to the intervention approach described in this book is that they provide an additional opportunity for students with CCNs to experience their language system within a real context. To create a visual schedule, begin by breaking down the student's day into individual steps, tasks, or activities. The degree of detail will depend on the individual needs of the student. Each step or activity is then visually represented and placed on a vertical laminated strip using Velcro. At the bottom of the visual schedule be sure to include a completion pocket with the symbol for "all done" clearly visible to the student. This is where the student will place the symbol of the completed activity in the "all done" pocket when they are done with that activity. Students are prompted to check their schedule with a consistently used verbal prompt (e.g., "check your schedule"), complete the activity or task at the top of their schedule, and return to their schedule upon completion to remove the picture icon and to place it in the "all done" pocket.

One of the purposes of using a visual schedule is to provide the student who is learning to communicate using a visually symbolic system an additional opportunity to experience their language system in action. Therefore, to enrich the language exposure opportunity, it is important to expand the visual representation of the activity or task. Instead of using a single symbol to represent a task or activity, take this opportunity to expose the student to core vocabulary and activity-related fringe words. For example, instead of having a single symbol representing "student on floor ready for circle time" use the symbols "sit," "on," and "floor" to express to the student to "sit on the floor."

> The benefits of visual schedules are often underestimated. In fact, some individuals feel that visual schedules feed into the student with autism's tendency toward rigidity. However, the converse is actually true. Visual schedules can actually be used to teach students to be more flexible and accepting of changes in their routines.

Students may have to be taught how to use a visual schedule. The picture symbols and the process of using a visual schedule may not be meaningful to the student at first, but with consistency and repetition, students will learn how to use them and demonstrate increased independence and calmness with their implementation (Bryan & Gast, 2000; Mesibov et al., 2002).

I Do, I Get

An "I do, I get" board is an example of a visual support that helps a student understand how much work they need to complete in order to earn a preferred item or activity. The "I do" side of the board, using a token system, provides a visual representation of how many trials or tasks the student must complete before earning what is visually represented on the "I get" side of the board. Upon completion of each trial or activity, the student earns a token that is placed on the board using Velcro in one of the spaces provided. The total number of spaces provided depends on how many trials or tasks you want the student to complete before earning their coveted reward. It is important to represent "I do" and "I get" as individual symbols for "I," "do," and "I," "get." These boards give the student with CCNs an opportunity to experience one way these core vocabulary words (i.e., I, do, get) can be applied.

Choice Boards

Choice boards are just that, a board with symbols of items and activities the student can choose from. Basically, it is a visual display of options. Choice boards are used for a variety of reasons, such as increasing a student's participation in circle time activities by allowing them to choose what song to sing or what book to read. Choice boards also allow students to self-determine what preferred activity or item they want to earn upon completion of a non-preferred task. Choice boards are customized based on the individual needs of the student and based on the purposes for what they are used. The purpose for which you will use a choice board will influence how you set it up. So that choice boards also serve the function of providing the student who is learning to communicate through the use of an AAC system an additional opportunity to be exposed to their language system, it is important to include symbols reflecting the purpose of the choice. Consider the following examples. Aligning with the intervention approach described in this book, be sure each word is represented as an individual symbol.

- ◆ "I-want-go" plus selection of places to go
- ◆ "I-want-watch" plus selection of movies or TV shows to watch
- ◆ "I-want-sing" plus selection of songs to sing during circle time
- ◆ "I-want-read" plus selection of books to read
- ◆ "I like" plus selection of preferred activities and items
- ◆ "I want wear" plus selection of clothes items
- ◆ "I-do-I-get" plus selection of preferred activities and items

Activity Scripts

As previously mentioned, comprehending oral language is very difficult for many of these students. Activity scripts are visual representations of different activities to support students with CCNs' participation, understanding, and attention in school-based events. Too often, students with CCNs are simply lost during classroom activities as they don't understand the expectations or what the next step is. Imagine if you had to participate in an environment in which you did not understand the language. This occurs for these students on a daily basis. Activity scripts provide the visual support these students need to make sense of their surroundings. Activity scripts can be created for a variety of activities including morning songs (e.g., "Hello Song") or craft activities. Obstacle courses are a great venue for introducing students to prepositions. An activity script composed of the symbol "go" and various prepositional symbols reinforces their understanding of prepositions. Visuals supports serve two purposes for the students described in this book: (1) increase comprehension and (2) expose students to their language system.

ACCESS TO LITERACY AS A MEANS TO FACILITATE COMMUNICATION AND LANGUAGE

Literacy, the ability to read and write (Beukelman & Mirenda, 2013), affords us many opportunities. In fact, it has been well established that early literacy opportunities, such as shared reading experiences, provide a cornerstone for the development of communication and language skills. Shared reading is an interactive reading experience in which young children with the guide and support of their teacher jointly share the reading of a big book or other enlarged text (Holdaway, 1979). In addition to being introduced to critical concepts of how print works, shared reading experiences give young children opportunities to engage in social communicative acts, such as asking and answering questions, as well as commenting and labeling for the purpose of sharing information. Shared reading interactions expose children to novel vocabulary and language within typical interactions. It is discouraging to consider that for many students with CCNs, the role literacy plays in supporting the development of communication is often underestimated or underutilized. In addition to having fewer literacy exposure opportunities, children with CCNs often do not engage in the same types of interactive book sharing exchanges as typically developing children (Light, Binger, & Kelford Smith, 1994; Light & Kelford Smith, 1993).

One barrier to a student with CCNs' access to children's literacy is that the language of stories can be too complex or abstract. The student with CCNs is learning to communicate through the use of picture symbols and the language of children's stories is based on oral and written language systems. Further hindering their access to the benefits of literacy is the fact that many children with CCNs experience impairments in motor skills that impede their ability to independently select a book off a shelf, position the book to the correct orientation, and manipulate the pages. It is imperative students with CCNs have access to shared reading experiences because they are missing valuable learning opportunities. For students with CCNs, shared reading experiences:

- Provide a venue to introduce new vocabulary
- Increase language exposure opportunities
- Teach multifunction word use
- Model question-response interactions
- Create communication opportunities
- Model more complex forms of language.

As previously introduced, *Adapted Stories*, a concept introduced by the author of this book, are books that are physically, linguistically and cognitively adapted to ensure children with CCNs have access to these language-enriched learning opportunities. Stories adjusted in this manner are not only physically accessible but also comprehensible to the student with CCNs. In the process of providing the student with CCNs opportunities to experience their language system, in this case picture symbols in print, adapted stores provide them with language models similar to those experienced by typically developing children during early literacy type of activities. Adapted stories provide a great platform for increasing students' symbolic knowledge by providing them with opportunities to observe how symbols can be used within context to convey meaning. Additionally, adapted stories support students' understanding of a story's content, and the ability to participate meaningfully in these types of learning experiences. Adapted stories can be used to introduce novel vocabulary and alternative uses of multiple meaning core vocabulary. It is through adapted stories that language can be modeled within context. Students learn how words and symbols are combined to convey meaning. What do adapted stories look like?

What Are Adapted Stories?

Adapted stories are stories that have been modified in a manner so they are manageable to the student with CCNs. That means they are presented in a language system that is comprehensible to the student at a level they can comprehend. Furthermore, books are physically modified so they are durable and easily manipulated by small hands or by those with physical challenges. How is that accomplished?

Physically Accessible

Many children with complex communication needs, including those with developmental delays and autism, experience fine motor challenges. Often viewed as "associated symptoms" in children with autism (Ming, Brinmacombe, & Wagner, 2007; Provost, Lopez, & Heimerl, 2007) and other diagnoses, fine motor deficits can hinder a student's ability to participate in a shared reading experience. Therefore, it is important books are physically modified so they are accessible to students with CCNs. This can be accomplished a variety of ways. Board books' and laminated pages are thicker, which can make it easier for those with fine motor difficulties to manipulate the page, and they are more durable, which allows them to withstand repetitive use. Page fluffers and turners can be added to provide students with a means to manipulate pages so they can become more actively involved in the reading experience.

> What are page fluffers and turners? Page fluffers and turners are physical adaptations that make turning pages for little hands, or for those who experience difficulty turning pages due to fine motor challenges, easier.

Linguistically Accessible

Students with CCNs are learning to communicate using a language system expressed in picture symbols. Adapted stories pair story text with picture symbols to allow the student who is developing communication skills through the use of picture symbols to experience their language system within the context of these stories. Representing story text in this manner not only models language concepts and use, but supports the student's comprehension of the content and supports their development of understanding the concept of a story. A causal benefit of supporting text with picture symbols is improvement in the students' attention to and participation in the story lesson. Too often students with CCNs are labeled as non-attentive or non-compliant during story time activities. Students with CCNs may become frustrated with having to listen to yet another story that does not make sense to them.

Cognitively Accessible

Because of delays in cognitive functioning, students with CCNs frequently struggle with the complexity of language presented in many children's stories, although the language of picture stories can be quite simple and frequently based on core vocabulary. *Gallop* by Rufus Butler Seder is an example of such a book. In this book, the repetitive phrase, "Can you *fly* like a *butterfly*?" is composed of the core vocabulary words "can," "you," and "like," with fringe words for animals and their associate action words. Conversely, there is a high percentage of children's literature in which the language is just too complex even to a point of abstractness. These stories require students to make causal connections, draw conclusions, and infer meaning. These are great skills to foster in typically developing children but for the student with CCNs this can be overwhelming and confusing. Further compounding the cognitive demands is the polarity between the story text and the illustrations. What is stated in the story text does not always coincide with graphics presented on the page. Children with comprehension difficulties rely heavily on the visual cues of the illustrations to make sense of the story. When the story text and illustrations don't match up, this strategy is lost. Adapted stories rework the story text so that is at the level of the student's abilities, taking advantage of the illustrations to support the student's understanding of the story's content.

What Are the Benefits of Adapted Stories?

In addition to the benefits of shared reading experiences previously outlined, using adapted stories for these types of interactions enhances the learning opportunities for students with CCNs.

◆ Adapted stories model language use within real contexts. They provide students with opportunities to observe how their language system can be used to ask questions, respond to questions, make comments, and share preferences within a structured but naturalistic dyad.

◆ Adapted stories provide multiple exposure opportunities to core vocabulary and other frequently used words. It has been well established that children begin to use words only after "hearing" them multiple times in everyday interactions within their environment (Harris & Reichle, 2004). Adapted stories are yet another opportunity to expose students to the symbols of their language system.

◆ Adapted stories introduce novel vocabulary often in a repetitive format. In addition to providing additional opportunities for students with CCNs to experience their vocabulary within the context of more naturalistic exchanges, children's literature often introduces thematic-based vocabulary in a repetitive format.

◆ Adapted stories support students' understanding of spoken language. Many students with CCNs experience great challenges understanding spoken language. The inclusion of picture symbols to supplement the story text provides the visual support necessary for them to gain a sense of the story. In some instances, story text may be simplified in order to make it more comprehensible. By pairing picture symbols with the simplified story, text stories are created that are understandable to the child, and expand their abilities to benefit from and participate in reading experiences.

◆ Adapted stories expand understanding of symbol knowledge. Within the context of a story, a student learns that symbols convey meaning and that symbols can be combined to express a variety of messages for an expanding range of communicative purposes such as requesting, commenting, and directing the behavior of another person. They learn multiword function use; that is, a single core vocabulary word can mean different things depending on how it is used or how it is paired with other words/symbols.

◆ Adapted stories can increase or improve a student's ability to use oral language. This is a beautiful thing! In many instances picture symbols cue children to use spoken language. It has been this author's experience that for a group of children who begin as functionally nonverbal (refer to Chapter 1 for a description of a functionally nonverbal student), picture symbols provide the necessary visual cues to support the output of oral language. With repetitive practice, picture symbols are gradually faded as the child uses increasingly more oral language. In cases such as these, we are able to methodically expand core vocabulary and introduce additional fringe vocabulary, including the incorporation of smaller words to expand the student's language structure patterns.

◆ Adapted stories provide students with additional communication opportunities. Within a shared reading experience or story lesson, the adult can scaffold a multitude of communication exchanges in which the child assumes both the role of initiator and responder. Opportunities to request and provide information, comment, and direct the next step are all possible within this context.

CREATING ADAPTED STORIES

Literacy experiences give students opportunities to practice using communication for a variety of communicative acts. including answering questions, labeling, and commenting. By adapting stories as suggested in this section, it is possible to create a language-enriched learning experience that is comprehensible to the student. It also gives communication guides a chance to scaffold interactive learning opportunities. The following is a list of steps to creating adaptive stories.

Step #1: Select a Book

The first step in creating an adapted story is to select a book. The language of early children's stories frequently reflects core and high-frequency fringe vocabulary (e.g., body parts, colors, clothing) because this is the language of young communicators. Although almost any picture book can be adapted, some books are more easily modified than others. Books with a repetitive word(s) or phrase(s) provide multiple exposure opportunities to reinforce students' learning of these key terms. For example, in the book *From Head to Toe* by Eric Carle, the phrases, "Can you do it?" and "I can do it!" are repeatedly used throughout the book, giving students multiple times to experience the use of these words within this question-response exchange. Appendix C provides a list of popular children's stories with repetitive phrases and suggests how these repetitive phrases can be altered using core vocabulary.

Step #2: Write a Story

Interactive literacy experiences expand children's language abilities by exposing them to more complex forms of language and novel concepts. However, the language used in stories for young children is often too complex and incomprehensible to students with CCNs. Therefore, it is sometimes necessary to adjust a story's language so that it is linguistically and cognitively accessible for them.

There are no fixed rules for adapting a story's text because each story is as unique as the needs of the students they are intended for. However, there are a few things to consider when modifying a story's text. As story text is rewritten, it is important to keep in mind the purposes of the modifications. They are (1) to ensure the story is understandable and (2) to increase students' opportunities to experience the language of their AAC system. In addition to increasing students' exposure opportunities to core vocabulary, adapted stories can support students' understanding of a story. A ratio of four core words to every fringe word is suggested. However, there are some stories in which this is not easily accomplished and there may be a greater concentration on fringe vocabulary. In these instances, the fringe vocabulary words introduced in the story have direct application to the emergent communicator. Stories that teach children about body parts and different kinds of food share value with those that introduce children to the variability and application of core vocabulary. Refer to Table 4–3 for examples of how story text is adapted using core vocabulary.

> Helpful Tip: Grab the sticky notes! Put sticky notes on each page you want to include in your story. When you go to make your picture symbols to match the story you created, it is easy to turn to each page in your story and see the picture symbols you need.

Another critical consideration in developing a story that is linguistically and cognitively accessible to a student with CCNs, is to match the story text to the picture. Children with CCNs frequently experience difficulty understanding oral language, and the presence of picture symbols often aids their understanding of the text. Visual cues in the illustrations are also important in supporting the students' understanding of the text. Because story books written for the typically developing child require them to make inferences based on text, and not on pictures alone, the adaptation of these for the child

Table 4–3. Examples of How to Modify Story Text

Picture Description	Story Text	Adapted Text
From *Head to Toe* by Eric Carle		
Picture of penguin	I am a penguin and I turn my head. Can you do it?	<u>Turn</u> <u>my</u> head. <u>You</u> <u>do</u> <u>it</u>? (or <u>Can</u> <u>you</u> <u>do</u> <u>it</u>?)
Picture of boy	I can do it!	<u>I</u> <u>do</u> <u>it</u>! (or <u>I</u> <u>can</u> <u>do</u> <u>it</u>!) Or <u>My</u> <u>Turn</u>!
Picture of a giraffe's body	I am a giraffe and I bend my neck. Can you do it?	Bend <u>my</u> neck <u>You</u> <u>do</u> <u>it</u>? (or <u>Can</u> <u>you</u> <u>do</u> <u>it</u>?)
Giraffe's head and boy	I can do it!	<u>I</u> <u>do</u> <u>it</u>! (or <u>I</u> <u>can</u> <u>do</u> <u>it</u>!) Or <u>My</u> <u>Turn</u>!
Where Is Maisy? by Lucy Cousins		
Text only	Is Maisy hiding in the house?	<u>Where</u> is Maisy?
Picture of a house	Not here	<u>Not here</u>!
Text only	Is Maisy hiding in the boat?	<u>Where</u> is Maisy?
Picture of a boat	Not here	<u>Not here</u>!
The Very Hungry Caterpillar by Eric Carle		
Caterpillar looking for some food	He started to look for some food.	Caterpillar feels hungry Caterpillar wants to eat
One apple	On Monday he ate through one apple but he was still hungry	Caterpillar eat one apple Caterpillar want more food Caterpillar feels hungry
Picture of chocolate cake	On Saturday he ate through one piece of cake, one ice cream cone, one pickle, one slice of Swiss cheese, one slice of salami. . . . That night he had a stomachache!	Eat more food (or I want eat more food) I feel bad

continues

Table 4–3. *continued*

Picture Description	Story Text	Adapted Text
Good Night Gorilla by Peggy Rathman		
Picture of Gorilla stealing keys from security guard	Good night, Gorilla	I get that!
Picture of Gorilla using the key to let the lion out of his cage. Security guard walking away	Good night, Lion	Come out, Don't tell

Carle, E. (1999). *From head to toe.* New York, NY: HarperCollins Publishers; Cousins, L. (1999). *Where Is Maisy?* London, UK: Walker Books Ltd; Carle, E. (1981). *The very hungry caterpillar.* New York, NY: Philomel Books; Rathman. P. (1994). *Good night gorilla.* New York, NY: G.P. Putnam's Sons Books for Young Readers.

with CNNs may be challenging. Try to pick stories in which the text and pictures match evenly or adjust the story text to correspond to the picture. Students with CCNs use visual cues present in a story's pictures to make sense of the story. When the text and accompanying picture do not match, it can create confusion for the individual with CCNs. Therefore, it is important that the story text represent what is being depicted in the picture.

> Helpful Tip: Include "all done" at the end of your story to provide additional opportunities for the student to see the concept of "all done" in action.

When modifying story text to meet the needs of the individual with CCNs, the following guidelines are helpful.

- Reserve the sense of story to the maximum extent possible.
- Write the story text to match illustrations.
- Balance the core and fringe vocabulary by striving for a 4:1 ratio of core words to fringe words.
- Capitalize on repetitive phrases.
- Use sentences and phrases three to five symbols in length as a general rule.

The primary goal of adapted stories is to provide students with CCNs repeated exposure to the symbols that comprise their communication system. Mastery of a strategically select set of words, core, and pertinent fringe vocabulary, can provide students with CCNs a means to communicate countless messages. As demonstrated in many of the examples provided in this chapter, and on the accompanying website, small words may be left out. Remember many of these children are emergent communicators and their language skills are consistent with a child at the one-to-three-word level in terms of the length and complexity of their utterances.

Select Your Picture Symbols

How story text is represented in symbols is as critical as the text itself. Ideally, the picture symbols used to represent the words in the story should reflect the symbol system used in the classroom (e.g., picture schedules) and in the student's AAC system, although there may be challenges with accomplishing this. For example, not all students in the classroom are using the same AAC language system. The most commonly used symbol sets are Picture Communication Symbols (PCS) by Boardmaker® and SymbolStix®, which is used by several popular apps.

Each word should be represented by its own symbol. Do not use a single symbol to represent a phrase or cluster of words. For example, "My turn" is depicted with the picture symbol "my" and the picture symbol representing "turn" situated side by side (Figure 4–8). This ensures that the student learns the individual identity of each word/symbol and how words/symbols can be combined with others words to convey different meaning (e.g., "my turn" "turn me").

Step #3: How to Build the Book?

The next step after adapting the story text and selecting the symbols, is to physically put the book together. The first goal is to ensure the book can be

> The only exceptions to this rule are the phrases "all done" and "thank you" that can be represented as single pictures.

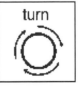

Figure 4–8. My Turn. The Picture Communication Symbols ©1981–2015 by Mayer-Johnson LLC, a Tobii Dynavox company. All Rights Reserved Worldwide. Used with permission. Boardmaker® is a trademark of Mayer-Johnson LLC.

manipulated by small hands or those with fine motor challenges. Secondly, it takes time to create these books, so you will want your books to physically withstand the wear and tear of repeated readings. How an adapted story is constructed will depend on how it will be used.

Type of Book

Big books are great for presenting a story to a group of students. Board book versions of stories can be more durable and frequently do not require as many physical adaptations in order to make them physically accessible. For books purchased in paperback form, it is recommended that pages be laminated so they can withstand repetitive use. Depending on the thickness of the lamination, it may be necessary to reinforce pages on cardstock. In order to accomplish this, it will be necessary to purchase two copies of the book because one side of the page will be covered up with the cardstock. Purchasing used versions of books (e.g., used book sites, amazon.com) or ordering books through the Scholastic Store (scholastic.com), which frequently offers popular children's stories at a low rate will help keep the costs down.

Affix Symbols to Pages of Story

Once you have printed out your picture symbols, affix them to the pages of your story. The question often arises, "Do you cover up the original text with the picture symbols?" The answer depends on how you will be using the book. If you will be reading the book to students with a wide range of abilities and intervention needs, it may be preferred to leave the text visible. Sometimes there is just not enough room on the page so you have no choice but to cover the text.

> If you are using a board book or do not have time to laminate the pages of your book, then clear packing tape is a great option to adhere the pictures to the pages and protects them from continual use. Leave at least a ¼-inch border around your symbols so they do not peel up.

Physical Adaptations

Physical adaptations such as incorporating page fluffers and flippers can also give students physical access to the story (Musselwhite & King-DeBaun, 1997). Page fluffers, also referred to as spacers, and page turners, are simple physical adaptations that can be added to make turning pages less difficult for those with fine motor challenges. Page fluffers create a gap between pages making it easier for little fingers to slip between pages. Page turners assist students who have difficulty turning pages. The following is a list of potential page fluffers and turners.

◆ Foam stickers
◆ Pom-poms (use a variety of sizes and stickers to create dimension to stories)
◆ Velcro pieces
◆ Makeup sponges
◆ Drop of glue from hot glue gun
◆ Paperclips (add beads to increase space and add color)
◆ Pieces of felt fabric
◆ Daily contact case covers
◆ Picture frame dots
◆ Chip clips
◆ Popsicle sticks
◆ Tongue depressors/craft sticks
◆ Buttons
◆ Bread closures
◆ Index tabs

Another option is to use clear, textured medical tape. In addition to reinforcing the pages for added durability from repetitive use, the texture of the tape makes grasping the laminated pages, which can be slippery, easier.

Step #4: Make Your Story Interactive

A variety of strategies are used to encourage children to participate in shared reading experiences. One strategy is for the adult to pause from time to time allowing the child to complete a sentence or recall a repetitive phrase that may occur throughout the story. This is a challenge for a student with CCNs. A single message output device (e.g., BIGmack communicator available from http://www.enablemart.com or http://www.ablenetinc.com) that is pre-recorded with a key phrase or word that frequently occurs during the story provides students with CCNs a means to participate in this manner. Every time the child sees a designated picture symbol, he or she activates the pre-recorded message. Another strategy used to facilitate children's participation in stories is asking them to identify pictures in the story or predict what a character might say or do. This too proves a challenge for children with CCNs. The PenFriend (available from a variety websites including http://www .indepedentliving.com and http://www.augresources.com) is an example of a voice labeling system in which messages are pre-recorded onto self-adhesive labels that can be strategically affixed to various pages throughout the story. As appropriate, the student can be prompted to activate the message by touching the tip of the PenFriend to the label. Strategies such as these provide students with CCNs opportunities to use communication in interactive types of experiences. Appendix D provides examples of popular children's stories and how they can be adapted physically, linguistically, and cognitively to meet the needs of students with CCNs.

TRAINING COMMUNICATION GUIDES

The success of the intervention approach described in this book is dependent on the skills of those implementing it. Speech-language pathologists, classroom teachers, instructional aides, speech-language pathology assistants (SLPAs), and graduate student interns are examples of those who may be recruited to assume the role of communication guide. Although the roles and responsibilities of communication guides will vary greatly, the primary role of the communication guide is to work one-on-one with the novice AAC user, guiding him or her through the communicative process and scaffolding communication opportunities and modeling AAC use. The expectations of the communication guides will influence how you structure your training sessions. For example, it is reasonable to expect that all communication guides will collect data on a daily basis and model AAC applying language stimulation techniques (e.g., self-talk, expansionism) and using aided modeling techniques. However, it might be the responsibility of the SLP or classroom teacher to develop goals and objectives. Regardless of these responsibilities, all communication guides need to understand the intervention process.

Communication is a dynamic, intrinsic process; therefore, it is important to begin the training by providing a brief description of AAC, including introduction of key terms related to AAC. Communication guides need to understand the complexity of AAC use. Light's (1989) model of communicative competence provides a framework for conceptualizing this. Understanding the range of purposes for which young communicators communicate will allow them to facilitate use of AAC for purposes beyond requesting preferred objects, food items, and routines. One of the overarching goals of the intervention described in this book is to teach novice AAC users how to use their AAC system for an expanding range of communicative purposes.

It is imperative to the intervention process described in this book that communication guides recognize the importance of teaching core vocabulary over fringe words. One way this can be introduced is to provide each communication guide with a communication board comprised primarily of fringe words, similar to the one in Figure 4–1. Then instruct the communication guides to create a list of two to three-symbol phrases they can formulate using the board in front of them. Then have them build a similar list of phrases based on a communication board of predominately core vocabulary words, similar to the one in Figure 4–2. Follow this up by discussing the types of communicative acts a student may need throughout their day.

Communication guides need to understand the complexities of communicative competence and how goals are developed across each of the competency areas. Discuss the importance of teaching core vocabulary and activity-specific fringe vocabulary. Also give them opportunities to develop skills to proficiently apply language intervention practices using aided modeling techniques. Help them understand how to teach communication through motor planning and how to create a language rich environment employing various visual strategies found effective in working with children with severe forms of autism and complex communication needs. Appendix A provides a detailed outline of the suggested topics to cover when training communication guides.

MOVING TO INTERVENTION IMPLEMENTATION

In the early stages of implementing the intervention, and until the student gains mastery of an expanding vocabulary, begin slowly by introducing one to two new words per activity. Select activities that will facilitate communication, focusing more on the process of the activity and less on the end product (e.g., craft). Sensory-based activities keep students engaged, which leads to better learning. Communication occurs all the time and it is not a pull-out service or rotation. Link everything the student does to a communication opportunity. Intervention teams have found it useful to use a "daily goal" matrix to ensure everyone knows how the student's communication goals can be facilitated throughout their day (Figure 4–9). Chapter 5 reviews how to implement an evidenced-based AAC intervention.

Communication: Daily Goal Matrix

Student's Name: J.M Goals: Insert Dates

Goal	Arrival	Toileting	Circle Time	Rotations	Snack	Recess	Rotations	O/T	Lunch	Story Time	Dismissal
*Use of 10 core and 15 fringe words. *Linguistic Competence*	X	X	X	X	X	X	X	X	X	X	X
*Construct 2-3 word/symbol messages. *Linguistic Competence*	X	X	X	X	X	X	X	X	X	X	X
Use communication system for no less than 3 different communicative purposes (e.g., request, greet peers/staff, protest). *Social Competence*	Greeting, assistance	Assistance, completion of task	Answer/ask questions, comment, request action	Varies across tasks	Request objects/actions, comment completion of snack	Request action/object, comment	Varies across tasks	Request recurrence, protest, assistance	Request objects/actions, comment completion of lunch	Answer/ask questions, comment, request action	Greeting, assistance
Demonstrate no less than 3 navigational skills (e.g., turn on, swipe, find/activate communication app, return to home, erase message). *Operational Competence*	X	X	X	X	X	X	X	X	X	X	X
Transition communication system to the next activity. *Operational Competence*	X	X	X	X	X	X	X	X	X	X	X
Demonstrate persistence by touching an adult on their shoulder to gain their attention and restate his message. *Strategic Competence*	X	X	X	X	X	X	X	X	X	X	X

Notes:
- *Target goals throughout J.M.s day.*
- *Continue to model use of communication for an expanding array of communicative functions.*
- *Model more complex forms of language using aided language-modeling strategies to employ language stimulation strategies such as self-talk and expansionism.*
- *Use least-to-most prompting hierarchy.*
- *Scaffold communication opportunities.*
- *Expect communication.... when not... model language use and form.*

*Refer to daily Communicative Competency Goals Daily Data Collection Form or Data Collection by Activity Form for specific words/symbols and phrases targeted per day and activity.

Figure 4–9. Daily Goal Matrix.

REFERENCES

American Speech-Language-Hearing Association (n.d.). *Augmentative and alternative communication.* Retrieved from http://www.asha.org/public/speech/disorders/AAC/#what_is

Banajee, M., DiCarlo, C., & Buras-Stricklin, S. (2003). Core vocabulary determination for toddlers. *Augmentative and Alternative Communication, 19*(2), 67–73.

Beukelman, D., Jones, R., & Rowan, M. (1989). Frequency of word usage by non-disabled peers in integrated preschool classrooms. *Augmentative and Alternative Communications, 5,* 243–248.

Beukelman, D. R., & Mirenda, P. (2013). *Augmentative and alternative communication: Supporting children and adults with complex communication needs* (4th ed.). Baltimore, MD: Paul H. Brookes.

Bryan, L., & Gast, D. (2000). Teaching on-task and on-schedule behaviors to high functioning children with autism via picture activity schedules. *Journal of Autism and Developmental Disorders, 30,* 553–567.

Fitzgerald, E. (1949). *Straight language for the deaf. A system of instruction for deaf children.* Washington, DC: AG Bell Association for the Deaf.

Harris, M., & Reichle, J. (2004). The impact of aided language stimulation on symbol comprehension and production in children with moderate cognitive disabilities. *American Journal of Speech-Language Pathology, 13,* 155–167.

Hill, K., & Romich, B. (n.d.) Core vocabulary and the AAC performance report. *Augmentative and Alternative Communication Institute.* Retrieved from http://www.aacinstitute.org/Resources/ProductsandServices/PeRT/CoreVocabularyAndTheAACPerformanceReport.html

Holdaway, D. (1979). *The foundations of literacy.* Sydney, Australia: Ashton Scholastic.

Light, J. (1989). Toward a definition of communicative competence for individuals using augmentative and alternative communication systems. *Augmentative and Alternative Communication, 5*(2), 137–144.

Light, J. (2003). Shattering the silence: Development of communicative competence by individuals who use AAC. In J. C. Light, D. R. Beukelman, & J. Reichle (Eds.), *Communicative competence for individuals who use AAC: From research to effective practice* (pp. 3–38). Baltimore, MD: Brookes.

Light, J. (2014). Communicative competence for individuals who require augmentative and alternative communication: A new definition for a new era of communication? *Augmentative and Alternative Communication, 30*(1), 1–18. http://dx.doi.org/10.3109/07434618.2014.885080

Light, J., Binger, C., & Kelford Smith, A. (1994). Story reading interactions between preschoolers who use AAC and their mothers. *Augmentative and Alternative Communication, 10,* 225–268.

Light, J., & Kelford Smith, A. (1993). The home literacy experiences of preschoolers who use augmentative communication systems and of their non-disabled peers. *Augmentative and Alternative Communication, 9,* 10–25.

Light, J., & McNaughton, D. (2014). Communicative competence for individuals who require augmentative and alternative communication: A new definition for a new era of communication? *Augmentative and Alternative Communication, 30*(1), 1–18.

Mesibov, G., Browder, D., & Kirkland, C. (2002). Using individualized schedules as a component of positive behavior support for students with developmental disabilities. *Journal of Positive Behavior Interventions, 25,* 58–72.

Ming, X., Brimacombe, M., & Wagner, G. C. (2007). Prevalence of motor impairment in autism spectrum disorders. *Brain and Development, 29*(9), 565–570.

Musselwhite, C. R., & King-DeBaun, P. (1997). *Emergent literacy success, merging technology and whole language.* Park City, UT: Creative Communicating Resources.

Provost, B., Lopez, B. R., & Heimerl, S. (2007). A comparison of motor delays in young children: Autism spectrum disorder, developmental delay, and developmental concerns. *Journal of Autism and Developmental Disorders, 37*(2), 321–328.

Van Tatenhoven, G. M. (2005). *Language functions and early generative language production.* Retrieved from http://homepage.mac.com/terryjohnmick/jafw/docs/aac_docs/NLDAAC.PDF

Tracy, B. (2007). *Eat that frog! 21 great ways to stop procrastinating and get more done in less time.* San Francisco, CA: Berrett-Koehler.

Wetherby, A. M., & Prutting, C. A. (1984). Profiles of communicative and cognitive-social abilities in autistic children. *Journal of Speech and Hearing Research, 27,* 364–377.

Wing, L., & Gould, J. (1979). Severe impairments of social interaction and associated abnormalities in children: Epidemiology and classification. *Journal of Autism and Developmental Disorders, 9*(1), 11–29.

Yorkston, K., & Karlan, G. (1986). Assessment procedures. In S. Blackstone (Ed.), *Augmentative communication: An introduction* (pp. 163–196). Rockville, MD: American Speech-Language-Hearing Association.

CHAPTER 5

Intervention Implementation Phase

Students with the most significant complex communication needs (CCNs) face profound challenges in developing even the most functional forms of communication. A myriad of interventions are often tried with these students with varying degrees of success. As these students progress through the educational system, they are often introduced to some type of augmentative and alternative communication (AAC) system, often without careful consideration of how they will be taught to use their AAC system. The intervention approach described in this book strategically plans intervention at the onset of assessment all the way through intervention implementation. Students with CCNs learn to communicate by being immersed in the language of their AAC system and by having opportunities to practice various skills associated with communication. The challenge is how to translate basic language intervention principles to teaching students to communicate through the use of AAC. The purpose of this chapter is to bridge AAC to evidence-based language intervention principles and practices.

Teaching a child to communicate through the use of AAC is less about being an "AAC Specialist" and more about being a good language therapist. It requires someone who possesses a breadth of knowledge of a wide range of evidence-based practices and who knows how to layer these various techniques and strategies to create an optimal learning environment in which language opportunities are created, participation is scaffolded, communication is expected, and AAC use is modeled.

The overarching goal of any AAC intervention is to improve AAC skills (Binger, Berens, Kent-Walsh, & Taylor, 2008). An AAC-based intervention approach not only promotes AAC skills, but facilitates acquisition of communication skills, supports a student's understanding of language (Goossens', 1989), and in many cases, promotes oral language (Harris & Reichle, 2004; Romski & Sevcik, 1996). Each child with CCNs presents with a unique set of challenges and strengths, thus, the intervention for these students must always be customized. It is for this reason so much time is devoted to the assessment and the intervention planning pieces of the intervention process described in this book. It is important we remind ourselves, and impart upon those who work with students who are learning to communicate through the use of an AAC system, that communication involves more than just requesting preferred food items and objects. Communication is a dynamic, multifaceted, fluid process. We must possess the expectation of communication from our students and assume they will learn to communicate for purposes that extend beyond requesting.

As intervention implementation is presented throughout this chapter, it will be important to remember that the intervention described in this book is not a specific technique but an approach that customizes the implementation of evidence-based practices to support a student in acquiring communication. Throughout this chapter, the concept of "layering" of techniques and strategies will be discussed. Intervention teams will need to use their own clinical judgement in deciding which evidence-based strategies will work best for their student, addressing their individual needs. Intervention is like a dance in which there is a fluid transition and mixture of techniques and strategies constantly in motion. An immersive environment is created, providing the student with an intensive intervention that capitalizes on social interactions. Table 5–1 provides an overview of the different techniques that are used to implement this intensive, immersive, socially based intervention.

INTENSIVE: SERVICE DELIVERY MODEL

Service delivery model refers to the manner in which related services—services provided to students who qualify for special education so that they may benefit from special education (Moore & Montgomery, 2017)—are provided to students with exceptional needs. An individualized educational program (IEP) specifies where a related service will be provided, who will be providing that service, and the duration or dosage of prescribed services (Cirrin et al., 2010). Pull-out, classroom-based, and indirect-consultative service delivery models are among the most common models prescribed by school-based speech-language pathologist to address the needs of students with a speech and/or language impairment.

One way that makes this intervention intensive is that it is provided in a prescribed block of time. In a public school setting, the most common service delivery model is pull-out, which is typically provided two to three times per week for sessions 30 minutes in length (Warren, Fey, & Yoder, 2007). With this type of service delivery model, students receive approximately 25 to 30 hours of intervention over the course of a school year. What if students received the identical amount of services in just two weeks? In order to help students firmly establish new skills, it is recommended students receive an intense

Table 5–1. Intensive, Immersive, Socially Based AAC Intervention

INTENSIVE (Service Delivery Model)	IMMERSIVE (Language Rich Environment)	SOCIAL (Communication Opportunities)
Block of Intervention	Communication Guides	Incidental Teaching
20 to 25 Hours of Intervention in 2 to 3 Weeks	Visual Supports	Child-Centered Approach
	Aided Modeling Techniques	Expectant Delay
	Language Stimulation Techniques	Communication Temptations
		Verbal Behavior
	Shared Reading Instruction	General Language-General Speech Pattern (GLGSP)
	General Language-General Speech Pattern (GLGSP)	

block of intervention over a period of two to three weeks. The goal is for students to receive 20 to 25 hours of intense intervention in a relatively short period of time. This can be accomplished in a variety of ways. These are a few examples of how services might be distributed over the course of two to three weeks:

◆ 2 hours, 5 days per week for 2 weeks (20 hours)
◆ 3 hours, 4 days per week for 2 weeks (24 hours)
◆ 4 hours, 3 days per week for 2 weeks (24 hours)

How it is written in an IEP will depend on how services will be provided. Consider writing total number of hours of services per month, semester, or year. Because of the many challenges these students face, follow-up sessions, either weekly, biweekly, or monthly, may be necessary to ensure they continue to develop their communication skills.

Will parents expect this type of intervention all day, every day? This has been a question posed by many administrators. This is an intense program. Students and communication guides are fatigued at the conclusion of each session every day. In fact, some students can only tolerate 2-hour blocks before becoming fatigued. At that point, the benefits are lost and negative behaviors are likely to increase. Engaging in negative behaviors is a way many of these students express a need for a break or change (*great opportunity to model a more appropriate response rate*). The best analogy I can give is to relate the intense intervention described in this chapter to attending an intensive sports camp or writing camp. At some point, you have to take what you have learned and practice it within your regular practices, games, or classes. The purpose of these intense camps is to firmly establish new skills so one can go back to their regular routines—in these examples weekly practices and games, or the classroom—and continue to reinforce and generalize these newly learned skills. At these intensive camps, an individual is hyper-focused on the execution of new skills. After developing a certain level of proficiency, they need to go back and simply practice these skills over and over within real contexts until they become automatic and the athlete or scholar no longer has to consciously think about how to execute them. A similar thought process applies here. Firmly establish new skills and then let the student return to their classroom and regular routines. One of the benefits of this type of intervention is to involve support staff from the student's regular classroom in the intervention so they become proficient in the techniques and strategies, so that they can continue to support the student when he or she returns to their regular classroom.

It may be challenging to carve out two to three hours, three to five times per week, for two to three weeks, for a multitude of reasons. Feel free to start small and gradually build your program. Bottom line: Doing something that is more intensive, immersive, and socially based is better than continuing with your current service delivery model. At one school, we started with an AAC Clinic one time per week for 45 minutes, gradually expanding to three times per week. At the middle school and high school levels, consider creating a communication class that students attend daily. Obviously, communication should not only be targeted during a specific class. However, it is necessary to devote time to teaching students new skills.

IMMERSIVE: LANGUAGE-RICH ENVIRONMENT

When we talk about placement options for students with language and communication disorders, we often use the term "language-based classroom." The benefits of a language-rich environment to the development of language and communication in young children has been well documented in the research, and is a fundamental element of any intervention program. A language-rich environment is created by adults modeling and giving children opportunities to experience their language within real contexts. Adults do this by talking to young children, modeling increasingly more complex forms of language. In language-rich classrooms children experience the language that poses them the greatest challenge through books and sensory activities. Children in language-based classrooms have multiple opportunities to practice using language. A language-rich environment immerses the child in the very language they are trying to learn. The confusion arises in how this looks in environments in which children are learning to communicate through the use of picture symbols and icons. How do we ensure they are being "immersed" in their language? What are the challenges and what are some of the solutions? Obviously, there is a disconnect between verbal language input and the expected output of students who are leaning to communicate through AAC.

We must figure out a way to create a language-rich environment consistent with the "language" we are trying to teach our students.

Communication Guides

This process begins by having a person who is knowledgeable and adept at using AAC intervention practices. It is well known that speech-language pathologists are the go-to professionals when it comes to teaching speech, language, and communication skills. However, to make the intervention described in this book effective, we must enlist the support of all professionals who interact with the student on a regular basis. These individuals must be versed in fundamental language intervention principles and know how they translate to AAC. Communication guides, as they are referred to as in this approach, continuously interact with the student who is learning AAC, creating communication opportunities and modeling language. Communication guides are often an extension of SLPs' expertise in language and communication, augmenting the richness of the intervention with their own unique skills and expertise. Communication guides will frequently find themselves in the role of communication partner, but their primary role is to create and scaffold communication opportunities between the student and their peers. Speech-language pathologists frequently serve as communication guides, but speech-language pathology assistants, school psychologists, teachers, instructional support staff, behavior therapists, and graduate student interns can all be trained to assume the role of communication guides. The author of this book frequently uses speech-language pathology graduate student interns as communication guides. Communication guides become the primary service provider during the course of the intervention. Appendix A provides a list of potential training topics to consider when training communication guides in preparation for implementation of intervention.

In order to implement the intervention model as it is intended, it is recommended that each novice AAC user be paired with a communication guide during the intervention sessions. For students who are more responsive to AAC intervention principles and/or are familiar with their AAC system, a higher student-to-adult ratio may be considered; however, in the initial stages of teaching a child to communicate via an AAC system a one-to-one ratio is preferred. A dedicated communication guide who will immerse the novice AAC user in the language of their communication system by applying various AAC strategies is essential to the intervention process. This is not to be interpreted that communication guides will be working one-on-one with the AAC user, but they are there to support the AAC user's participation in socially based activities.

As mentioned in Chapter 2, one of the adjunct benefits of this type of service delivery model is that it can be used to train support staff in how to implement AAC-based interventions. Support staff, after being properly trained, are coached and receive guided practice learning to implement best practices working with students with CCNs. At the end of the two weeks, they are ready to return with their student(s) back to their regular classrooms where they can continue to facilitate the student's use of their AAC system. As previously mentioned, this intervention model was initially developed as a training model for graduate speech-language pathology student interns, and has evolved into an evidence-based intervention model. It has since been used to train instructional aides in using effective strategies with students who use AAC.

Visual Supports

Students who are learning to communicate through the use of AAC need multiple opportunities to experience their language system in action. One way this can be accomplished is through the use of visual supports. Several examples, including adapted stories, and visual schedules, were discussed in Chapter 4. Consider other opportunities in which oral language can be paired with symbols reflective of the student's AAC system. The ultimate goal is to strive to pair verbal language models with the language of the student's AAC system. Every time verbal directions are given to the student with CCNs is an opportunity to expose that student to the language of their AAC system. Tables 5–2 and 5–3 provide examples of how visual supports can be developed to support a student's understanding of oral language, while simultane-

Table 5–2. Yoga Practices Teach Core Vocabulary "Do," and Prepositions Along with Body Parts

Yoga		
Yoga Move	*Directive*	*Language/Symbol Models*
Tree	Do Tree	Hands together Arms up Foot on leg
Downward dog	Do Downward dog	Bend body Hands on floor
Star	Do Star	Arms out Legs out
Fish	Do Fish	Lie on floor Chin up

Table 5–3. Obstacle Courses Teach Core Vocabulary, Including Action Words and Prepositions

Obstacle Course	
Obstacle	*Language/Symbol Models*
Tunnel	Go through
Stairs	Go up
	Go down
Hula-Hoop	Jump in
	Jump out
Ladder	Go up
	Go down
Jump rope	Go over
	Go under
Bean bag	Throw in
	Take out
	Put on head—walk
Ball and Bowling pin	Roll ball
	Knock down pins
	Put pins up

ously exposing them to the language of their system. A yoga activity can be used to give students experience with the core vocabulary "do," and prepositions along with body parts. An obstacle course can expose a student to core vocabulary words, including action words such as "go," "jump," "take," and "put," as well as preposition words. Later in this chapter we will continue this discussion of visual support including how to implement adapted books through shared reading experiences, and other visual supports in authentic contexts using aided modeling techniques.

Aided Modeling Techniques

Modeling, which is influenced by the social learning theory, is an intervention technique that gives language-delayed children an opportunity to "hear" targeted language structures without the demands of imitation. Providing rich language models is easily accomplished when the models are oral language. The challenge is how does this translate to an AAC intervention?

Aided modeling techniques, such as aided language stimulation (ALgS) and augmented input, encapsulate the intervention practice of pairing oral language models with picture symbols for the purposes of promoting the acquisition of communication and supporting the understanding of language (Binger & Light, 2007; Goossens', 1989; Romski & Sevcik, 2003). Coupling language modeling techniques and child-centered approaches through the application of aided modeling techniques provide students with CCNs opportunities to experience communication within naturalistic contexts.

Aided language stimulation (ALgS), as an example of an aided modeling technique, is a language stimulation practice in which the facilitator (e.g., teacher) uses the targeted AAC device in conjunction with oral language stimulation (Beukelman & Mirenda, 2013; Cafiero, 1998; Goossens', 1989). ALgS was initially introduced by Carol Goossens' in 1989 and has demonstrated positive effects in increasing a child's use of pictorial symbols, along with supporting their understanding of spoken language. A facilitating adult models the AAC use of picture symbols by pointing to picture symbols either directly on a student's communication system or other available pictures while talking. This approach teaches a child through modeling how to use picture symbols as a form of communication.

What does research tell us about the effectiveness of such techniques in helping students learn to communicate through the use of AAC? Although the research is still in the infancy stage, with a majority of studies reported being based on single case studies, the evidence is mounting to the success of its use with students who are learning to use AAC. Adults with developmental delays have shown increased use and responsiveness (Beck, Stoner, & Dennis, 2009), along with improved grammar (Lund & Light, 2003) when aided modeling techniques were used. In young AAC users, AAC modeling has shown promise as an intervention technique in teaching grammatical morphemes (Binger, Maguire-Marshall, & Kent-Walsh, 2011), and improving syntactic performance (Bruno & Trembath, 2006). Improved comprehension of vocabulary (Dada & Alant, 2009), along with improving symbol comprehension and production (Harris & Reichle, 2004), are additional benefits that have been observed when such techniques are used. Increased use of action-object messages (Nigam, Schlosser, & Lloyd, 2006) and multisymbol messages (Binger & Light, 2007) have also been document as one of the benefits of aided modeling techniques. Table 5–4 provides a brief description of the different aided modeling techniques, and provides relevant research to support their use.

In order for aided modeling techniques to be effective, they need to be applied during 70% of interactions (Dada & Alant, 2009). It is also recommended communication guides model comments (e.g., "I like blue," "I go") at a higher rate of frequency relative to questions, targeting a ratio of four comments to every question (Dada & Alant). In the end, aided modeling

Table 5–4. Aided Modeling Techniques

Aided Modeling Technique	Definition	Research
Partner Augmented Input	The term used by Dynavox to collectively refer to Aided Language Stimulation, Aided Language Modeling, and System for Augmenting Language (Senner, 2008).	
Aided Language Stimulation (ALgS)	Aided language stimulation provides the novice AAC user with both verbal and visual input. The facilitating adult pairs their oral language models with symbols on the AAC user's communication system. As the facilitating adult interacts with the individual who is learning to use AAC, he/she points to symbols on the AAC user's communication system that corresponds to their oral language models (Beukelman & Mirenda, 2013; Goossens', 1989)	Increases recognition and use of new symbols (Dada & Alant, 2009) Improves ability to compose messages that are more syntactically complex (Bruno & Trembath, 2006) Increases the number of communicative turns taken during group activities (Beck, Stoner, & Dennis, 2009) Parents increase use of basic ALgS techniques with their children at home during daily activities (Jonsson, Kristoffersson, Ferm, & Thunberg, 2011).
Aided Language Modeling (ALM)	While engaging in activities that are highly motivating to the student the facilitating adult pairs oral language with symbols. The facilitating adult draws the AAC user's attention to an object in the environment by pointing; while simultaneously saying the object label they point to a corresponding symbol. The facilitating adult can point to symbols directly on the AAC user's device but it is not necessary in this approach (Beukelman & Mirenda, 2013).	Increases symbol comprehension and production (Drager et al., 2006) Increases production of multi-symbol messages (Binger & Light, 2007) Parents and educational assistants increase use of ALM strategies with their children, resulting in acquisition of new communication and language skills (Kent-Walsh & McNaughton, 2005).

continues

Table 5–4. *continued*

Aided Modeling Technique	Definition	Research
System for Augmenting Language (SAL)	In this technique the facilitating adult activates symbols on a speech-generating device (SGD) to augment their speech input. In essence, the individual receives input from three sources: the speech of the facilitating adult, output of the SGD, and the symbol on the device itself. The facilitating adult may only point to key symbols during the interaction as a means to highlight key words (Beukelman & Mirenda, 2013).	Increases use of symbols in combination with gestures and vocalizations to serve various communicative functions including to request items, assistance, and information, to comment, and to answer questions (Romski & Sevcik, 1996)
		Increases use of meaningful and functional symbol combinations (Wilkinson, Romski, & Sevcik, 1994)
		Improves recognition of printed words displayed with symbols and increases intelligible spoken word productions (Romski & Sevcik, 1996)
		Conveys more conversationally appropriate, less ambiguous, and more specific information to an unfamiliar communication partner (Romski, Sevcik, & Adamson, 1999)

techniques provide students with CCNs with multiple opportunities to experience the vocabulary and language of their communication system, increasing students' comprehension and familiarity with the symbols that comprise their communication system (Harris & Reichle, 2004). Research has shown improved understanding of spoken language when oral language is paired with symbols (Goossens', 1989). An indirect benefit of aided modeling techniques is the positive impact it has on a student's use of oral language (Harris & Reichle, 2004; Romski & Sevcik, 1996). Many students who are routinely exposed to aided language modeling begin using oral language. Overall, aided modeling techniques provide students with greater opportunities to communicate (Cafiero, 1998).

> For maximum effect, aided modeling techniques should be applied during 70% of interactions

Language Stimulation Techniques

The application of indirect language stimulation techniques (Paul & Norbury, 2012), a hallmark feature of many early intervention programs, supports the young child in developing language and communication skills. Early interventionists, along with speech-language pathologists and parents, create a language-rich environment for the language-delayed toddler by providing a dialogue of their own actions (e.g., "I am pouring juice in the cup."), narrating the actions of the young child (e.g., "You are making the plane go up."), expanding on the child's communication attempts (e.g., child says, "car"; adult responds, "That is a big black car."), and modeling more complex forms of language. This seemingly naturalistic intervention approach is somehow lost in translation in its presentation to an individual who is learning to communicate through the use of AAC. There is a noted decrease in the number of oral language models provided to the emergent AAC user, as the adult questions the value of such experiences to a student who experiences such significant challenges understanding oral language models. Due to the child's limited response to the adult's language model, there is a gradual decrease in the number of oral language models provided to the child. The question arises, how do indirect language intervention techniques translate to AAC-based interventions? The answer is through the use of aided modeling techniques.

As previously discussed, the communication guide creates a language-rich environment by pairing oral language models with picture symbols. This gives the AAC user an opportunity to experience communication, specifically their communication system, within naturalistic contexts. The main challenge here is the language facilitator, in this case referred to as the communication guide, is restricted to the available picture symbols on the student's communication system. This illustrates the importance of providing the student with the maximum number of symbols on their communication board that they can possibly or potentially manage. A communication guide working with a student who has a communication board consisting of only four symbols will be significantly restricted in the number and type of language exposure opportunities they can provide to the emergent communicator. In instances when a child can only manage a small symbol set (e.g., 2 to 8 symbols), the communication guide has a couple of options. One option is to begin with a larger symbol set (e.g., 25 symbols) and cover up symbols that are not relevant to the current activity. The strategy of hiding icons is discussed later in this chapter. Another option is to use what is referred to as a *modeling board*. A modeling board is a communication board used by the communication guide to model communication opportunities and more complex forms of communication. The following is a brief description of the different indirect language stimulation techniques that can be used.

Self-Talk

Self-talk is an indirect language stimulation technique in which the facilitator or communication guide describes his or her own actions as he or she engages in parallel play with the student. In this approach, the communication guide talks about what he or she doing while the student is watching. Considered an effective intervention strategy for children between 12 to 24 months of age, it can be extremely effective for emergent communicators who are resistant to clinician-directed approaches (e.g., drill type therapy approaches). In this approach, the communication guide uses simple phrases to expose the student to novel language structures (e.g., action-object-location), while simultaneously demonstrating language use. The communication guide pairs self-talk with ALgS to reinforce use of the targeted device. The example provided in the text box illustrates how self-talk can be used without pressuring the emergent communicator to respond. In this instance, the communion guide provided multiple opportunities for the student to witness the use of core vocabulary words (i.e., I, have, open, want, my, no, more, did, it, get, all gone, need) for a variety of communicative purposes (e.g., requesting, commenting). As the child is repeatedly exposed to this scripted routine, the communication guide will gradually scaffold communication opportunities for the emergent AAC user to use their communication system. But in the beginning, the sole role of the AAC user is to enjoy the interaction and being exposed to the language of their communication system.

> While playing with bubbles, the communication guide might express the following phrases, pairing oral language models while simultaneously pointing to symbols on the student's communication system. Note core vocabulary words are bolded. **I have** bubbles, **I like** bubbles, **I want open** bubbles, **My** bubbles, **open** bubbles, Bubbles **no open**, **I turn**, **no open**, **more turn**, **I open** bubbles, **I do/did it**, I blow bubbles, **My** bubbles **go up**, **I get it**, **My** bubbles **all gone**, **I need more** bubbles, **I do it again.**

Parallel Talk

Parallel talk is an indirect language stimulation technique in which the communication guide provides a running description of the student's actions. This strategy provides a language model for the child to internalize (Paul & Norbury, 2012). Utilizing this strategy, the communication guide describes what the student is hearing, seeing, and doing. It is not necessary to comment on the student's every action as this can become overwhelming for the student. However, it is important to select a few key language structures and to target and focus on those. Repetition of these key language structures or phrases is good for the student and helps them recognize the language patterns and their functions within the given context. Parallel talk is provided utilizing ALgS.

You have truck

You have big red truck.

Truck go fast.

Truck stop.

Boy go in truck.

You make truck go fast

Description

Description is an indirect language stimulation technique in which the communication guide labels objects the student is playing with or sees. This is an excellent opportunity to introduce fringe vocabulary related to preferred objects and activities along with classroom objects. The student witnesses how attributes (e.g., colors, size) are paired with object symbols to describe and differentiate between objects. If the student demonstrates interest in a car, the communication guide may make reference to the car's color or size or even comment about the number of wheels on the car. Likewise, if a student demonstrates interest in a particular animal, in addition to referencing attributes to describe the animal the communication guide can use the action words that are typical of that particular animal.

> With experience, communication guides quickly blend parallel talk and description to create fluid language exposure opportunities.

Expansions and Recasts

Expansions is an indirect language stimulation technique in which the communication guide repeats the child's utterance, adding additional words or phrases creating a more semantically or syntactically complete utterance. The communication guide repeats the child's production and adds symbols to the child's initial message to create a more syntactically complete message. Comparatively, recasts is an indirect language stimulation technique in which the student's utterance is expanded into a different type of sentence, such as when a comment is expanded into a question.

EXAMPLE 1–Expansion: The communication guide expands on the student's use of a single symbol ("car") to request a car, to which the facilitating adult expands on the student's utterance by stating, "*I understand you want car . . . more language is* 'I want blue car,'" while simultaneously pointing to corresponding symbols on the student's communication system.

EXAMPLE 2–Expansion: In response to the student's communication attempt, "go," the communication guide expands this communication attempt using the General Language-General Speech Program (GLGSP), "*I understand you want me to make car go . . . your language is* 'Make car go.'"

Student: "I want blue car."

EXAMPLE 3–Recast: Communication Guide recasts as a question, "Does the blue car go fast?"

Although not considered a requirement of indirect language stimulation techniques, there is a high probability that the student will imitate, if not the entire phrase, at least part of the more complete utterance (Scherer & Olswang, 1984). Any attempt to practice these more complex utterances should be viewed as additional practice opportunities that inevitably help the student progress toward greater levels of communicative competence.

Shared Reading Instruction

In Chapter 4, we discussed how to adapt books (Dodd, 2011) so they were physically, linguistically, and cognitively manageable to the student with CCNs. In this section we discuss how to implement shared reading using these adapted stories. Shared reading, initially introduced by Don Holdaway in 1979, is a collaborative learning experience that occurs between the teacher and his/her students. In this interactive reading experience, students, with the support of a teacher, "share" in the reading of books (http://reading rockets.org). These types of interactions encourage students to be actively involved in the learning process. In the end, the interaction is viewed less as an instructional lesson and more as a shared event (Holdaway, 1979) in which the teacher intentionally encourages and supports the student's engagement and participation (Justice & Pence, 2005). In a typical shared reading model, the first reading is purely for enjoyment. During the second reading of the story, young children build and extend their comprehension of the story. The teacher may focus children's attention to the interesting language and vocabulary. By the fourth or fifth reading of the story, children start to decode words based on familiarity of the text and predictability (Yaden, 1989). For the child with CCNs, shared reading strategies are modified to give students multiple opportunities to experience the language of their AAC system, and provide opportunities and venues to introduce new vocabulary. Shared reading experiences give students naturalistic opportunities to participate and gain experience in answering and asking questions. As previously stated in Chapter 4, typical children's literature is often very complicated and difficult for a student with CCNs. Story text that is paired with picture symbols is more manageable and understandable to the child with CCNs as it helps them gain a sense of a story. Shared reading experiences provide an opportunity to expose students to more complex forms of communication. Table 5–5 briefly provides commonly used shared reading strategies and how they can be modified to use with students who are learning to communicate through the use of AAC.

General Language-General Speech Pattern (GLGSP)

Students with CCNs learn to use their communication system and become better communicators by having opportunities to experience and practice the act of communicating. A technique the author has used throughout her career in working with children with speech and language disorders, and has applied to her work with students with CCNs, is the General Language-General Speech Pattern (GLGSP) (Skatvold, 1976,). GLGSP was initially developed by Marguerite Stoner, based on her work with children who were deaf or hard of hearing at the John Tracy Clinic in Los Angeles, California, in the 1970s. It was later adapted by Elaine Ogle in the Irvine Unified School District for application with preschool-aged children with moderate to severe speech and language delays and disorders. GLGSP has been modified for its application with students who are learning to communicate through the use of an AAC system. So what is GLGSP and how does it apply to students who are learning to communicate through the use of AAC?

The GLGSP is a nonintrusive technique for cueing and modeling language in terms of form and function. As Skatvold (1976) stated, "GLGSP gives the child consistent, clear, and immediate feedback on the effectiveness of his (her) communication" (p. 191). Those who use GLGSP—communication partners, teachers, clinicians, and parents—continuously model language that is slightly above the child's current level of functioning, demonstrating for the child how they can use language in the moment. This later piece, experiencing how language can be used in the moment, is significant for students with CCNs. GLGSP gradually transitions the student with CCNs from being dependent on the adult's model of language to self-correcting or self-generating more appropriate forms of language. In the beginning the child may be completely dependent on the adult's model of language. Initially, or in novel situations, it may be necessary for the communication guide to provide the emergent AAC user with the specific language to use in the given situation. For example, consider a child who has had little experience or success in engaging in reciprocal type activities such as playing board or tabletop games.

Table 5–5. Shared Reading Strategies Applied to Students with CCNs

Share Reading Strategy	Description	AAC Implementation	Implementation
Picture Walk	A picture walk is a shared reading activity in which the facilitating adult previews the story with the child or group of children before actually reading the unfamiliar story. It has proven particularly beneficial to children who have difficulty simultaneously integrating multiple sources of information.	Previews a Story Introduces novel vocabulary words Asks questions to elicit target words	As the adult presents the story they can introduce the book upside down and model for the students on their AAC system "turn" or "turn it" to instruct the adult to turn the book to the correct orientation. Next, the adult models "open," "open it," or "open book" to introduce the students to the pages of the book. Throughout the picture walk, the adult models (and may even employ hand-over-hand modeling) "turn," "turn it," "more turn," "you turn," "I turn," or "turn page" to demonstrate to the student(s) how to direct the adult to turn pages. The facilitating adult asks students who, what, where, when, why, and how questions about the pictures. Sample questions include: "What is the boy doing?" "How do you think the dog feels?" "Where do you think the man is going?" "Why do you think the girl looks so excited?" and "What do you think will happen next?" The facilitating adult balances asking question to expand AAC use, use of core vocabulary, and increased communication opportunities.
Echo Reading	Echo reading is a shared reading strategy in which children echo or repeat what the facilitating adult is reading. Echo reading develops expressive language skills and facilitates fluent reading.	Repeats target words after teacher Repeats target phrases after teacher	As the facilitating adult reads the story, he/she models, using hand-over-hand prompting if necessary, key or repetitive phrases from the story. This gives students an opportunity to practice the language of the book so that during subsequent readings of the same story, students are familiar with not only the vocabulary or language of the story but the location of specific vocabulary and how to sequence symbols into meaningful phrases or sentences.

Strategy	Description	Features	Notes
Repeated Readings	Repeated readings is a fundamental characteristic of shared reading instruction. Children become increasingly more actively involved in the reading of a story following multiple exposures (Yaden, 1989). Through repeated readings and predictable text that is characteristic of early literacy books, children become familiar with word forms and begin to recognize words and phrases and begin to "read" the stories.	Reinforces vocabulary Multiple exposure opportunities Repetitive practice to mastery	The adult reads the same story over the course a week, or two weeks, giving the student multiple exposure opportunities to the vocabulary and language presented in the story.
Fill-in gap	Fill-in the gap is a shared reading strategy in which the facilitating adult pauses while reading the story with the expectation that the students will fill in the missing word or phrase.	Elicits target words Elicits target phrases	This strategy works really well with stories that have repetitive phrases or rely on a parallel language. This gives emergent AAC users an opportunity to participate in the telling of the story. It is important to target words or phrases consisting of core vocabulary and functional fringe words, such as colors or body parts. The more opportunities students have to practice using these words during engaging activities, the greater likelihood they will use them across environments and activities.
Extension Activities	The purpose of extension activities is to reinforce key vocabulary or concepts introduced in the story.	Acting out story with props Activities to reinforce vocabulary Activities to reinforce concepts Story sequencing activity	Extension activities will be developed based on the needs of the students.

In these instances, the communication guide models language that is suitable for the student to use in the current activity. For example, given a tabletop board game, the communication guide models applicable language to requesting a turn ("Your language is 'I want turn'"). The communication guide layers aided modeling techniques by simultaneously pointing to corresponding symbols on the student's AAC system as he or she provides the student with the relevant language models. As the child progresses and becomes more proficient in using their communication system, the communication partner fades their level of prompting to simply providing a verbal cue for the child to use their language or to use more language (e.g., "Use more language."). By providing the child with the simple verbal cue, "Use better language," they begin self-correcting their erred utterances and respond with ones that are more accurate. For example, a child says, "Where you go?" The facilitating adult responds, "Use better language," to which the child responds, "Where are you going?" Yes, it is that simple!

So how do you implement GLGSP with students who are learning to communicate through the use of AAC? The following is a summary of four steps to implementing GLGSP with students who are learning to communicate with the support of an AAC system. The GLGSP approach is a fluid process; A seamless flow of validating the student's communication attempts, evaluating their responses, and modeling or prompting accordingly all within the premise that in order to get a student to communicate we must expect that they will communicate.

STEP 1: Expect Communication

The first step to implementing GLGSP is to expect communication. It is important that communication guides not only expect that students will communicate, but that they will communicate for purposes that extend beyond requesting preferred food, items, and activities. If we think that students with the most complex communication needs are only capable of learning to communicate to control their immediate environment, then that is all we will teach them to do. Conversely, if we set the expectation that our students can and will learn to communicate for a wide range of communicative purposes, then we have exponentially increased the likelihood that this will occur. Additionally, the expectancy of communication must be equivalent across environments and communication partners. Therefore, communication among interested parties, including clinicians, teachers, parents, and support staff is critical so everyone who the student encounters on a daily basis has similar expectations for communication.

STEP 2: Validate Communication Attempt

Before prompting the student to use better or more language, or providing the student with an improved language model, it is important to validate the student's communication attempt. This confirmation lets the student know that his or her communication attempt has value. Children whose communication attempts are validated are motivated to try again. This can be accomplished by simply stating, "I understand." For example, consider a child who is pointing at a container of Cheese Balls on the shelf. The communication guide responds by stating, "I understand you want Cheese Balls. Your language is 'Want Cheese Balls,'" simultaneously pointing to symbols on the student's AAC system. In instances when the child's communication attempt is sufficient and relevant to the situation, the communication guide validates that by stating, "Good language, I understand" and then applies various language stimulation models such as expansionism or recasting applying GLGSP cueing as appropriate. In the event you do not understand, it would be appropriate to say, "I don't understand" and then provide the student with scaffolds to assist them in communicating their message.

STEP 3: Evaluate the Communication Attempt

The third step is to evaluate the student's communication attempt in terms of both form and function. All communication attempts are accepted and evaluated in terms of appropriateness and effectiveness. At this point, the communication guide, who knows the child well, evaluates the means in which the student delivered the message. If the student uses behavioral forms of communication, then the communication partner will model more socially appropriate forms of communication. Consider the following example in which the communication guide utilizes the communication temptation of providing the student with a non-preferred food item. The student responds by pushing the item away or even perhaps throwing it. The communication guide recognizes that this is not an appropriate or acceptable form of communication, although the student did convey his/her distain of the offered item, and models or prompts a more socially acceptable means of communicating. The exact model or prompt will be based on what he or she knows the student is capable of doing.

Of critical importance to evaluating the student's communication attempts is to continuously evaluate the purposes for which the student is communicating, and identify if there is an opportunity to demonstrate for them how to use their language in the given situation. These are the opportunities that demonstrate for the student how to use their AAC system for a range of communitive purposes including commenting ("I like it."), expressing emotions ("I feel mad."), requesting assistance ("I need help."), and sharing preferences ("No like.").

STEP 4: Model or Prompt Language

The last step is to elicit the appropriate response by either providing a model of the language you expect them to use or expanding on their communication

Table 5–6. General Language General Speech Program Prompts

Dependent Child	Independent Child
Your language is . . .	Use your language
More language is . . .	Use more language
Better language is . . .	Use better language

attempts. For your example you would say, "I understand you want a turn (validate communication attempt). Your language is . . . 'my turn.'" To a child who points to a single icon you would respond, "I understand you want me to open it." Your language is 'you open it.'" This exchange occurs simultaneously while the communication partner is applying aided modeling techniques. Table 5–6 provides a list of language prompts to use, depending on the needs of the student.

> One reason GLGSP is so effective is "the response at the end of the GLGSP is the positive reinforcement" (Skatvoid, 1976, p. 192).

SOCIAL: COMMUNICATION OPPORTUNITIES

One of the principal goals that must be accomplished for this intervention program to be successful is the creation of meaningful communication opportunities. This can be accomplished by strategically implementing specific techniques that give students opportunities to practice using their AAC system in socially engaging and motivating interactions. How we teach communication to students with CCNs will have a direct impact on their receptiveness to corrective feedback and ongoing instruction. Students need to associate communication with all its positive benefits, increasing their motivation to participate in the interaction. It is important to create a supportive environment that encourages all types of communication attempts, while shaping communicative acts into more socially acceptable and easily recognizable forms of communication. Both explicit instruction and incidental teaching contribute to teaching a student to use their AAC system (Beukelman & Mirenda, 2013). **Explicit instruction**, which is characteristic of interventions based on the principles of applied behavior analysis, consists of repeated trials of a targeted skill or behavior to the criterion level of mastery. A trial, which is repeated while prompts are faded, typically includes a stimulus, a prompt, elicitation of target behavior or skill, and delivery of a reinforcer (Beukelman &

Mirenda, 2013). The limitation of this type of teaching is it is often too far removed from the context of the actual skill. Additionally, the redundancy of the trials may, in turn, elicit negative behaviors from the student in an attempt to escape the unpleasant learning situation, decreasing their motivation to actively participate in similar learning dyads in the future. **Incidental teaching**, which shares many similarities to explicit instruction (e.g., stimulus, response, reinforcer), takes advantage of teachable moments, as well as methodically orchestrated communication opportunities to give students the practice they need to gain mastery of new skills. Child-centered approach, communication temptations, expectant delay, and verbal behavior are examples of incidental teaching approaches that will be discussed later in this chapter. Collectively, these intervention practices provide students with CCNs multiple opportunities to use their AAC system in functional, meaningful interactions.

Child-Centered Approach

A student's motivation and level of engagement in a learning activity will directly affect their response in a negative or positive manner. In the event a student is not engaged in the learning activity at hand, find out what they are interested in and center instruction and communication opportunities around that. One way to ensure a child is engaged in the learning process is to adopt a child-centered approach. For example, you discover midway through an activity a student is completely disengaged, but you recognize that one of the materials associated with the activity is highly motivating. You quickly turn this activity into a turn-taking interaction in which you and the student take turns playing with this item of interest. The student is using their communication system, you realize opportunities to model higher forms of language, and the student is engaged and enjoying the interaction. Win-win for everyone! It is more important the student is engaged in the process and not forced to participate is some prescribed activity.

Expectant Delay

Expectant delays provide the student ample time to process and respond to a communication guide's bid for interaction (Binger et al., 2008). This can be a difficult technique to practice because most individuals have an innate desire to keep a conversation going or to help the student by providing them with the language they need. We are too quick to help the student. Always give the student ample time to respond. Sometimes just waiting will serve as a prompt to the student he/she needs to do something to participate. Many of these students have learned passivity simply because they have not been given a chance to respond in their own time. For some of these students, processing what is being asked of them and then actually planning and executing a response takes time. Bottom line: don't be too quick to help these students out, give them time so they can contribute in their own way.

Communication Temptations

One of the most effective ways to "entice" a student to communicate is to use communication temptations. What are communication temptations? Communication temptations, as they are commonly referred to today, were initially introduced as "communicative situations" by Wetherby and Prutting (1984) in their research examining the communication and cognitive-social profiles of children with autism who were functioning at the pre-linguistic stages of language development. These communicative situations were developed as a method to tempt the child into initiating communication for purposes of gaining access to items of interest. Table 5–7 provides examples of various communication temptations and the types of communication functions typically evoked by each, and what potential language communication guides can expect from their students or model for them. It is important to recognize that communication temptations elicit communication primarily for the purposes of regulating the behaviors of others for the purposes of gaining access to preferred food items, activities, or actions. Therefore, communication guides need to be cognizant of that and be thinking of how they can adjust their interaction to elicit other communicative functions.

Communication Temptations–Desired food item in closed container, Necessary item: A student says, "I want fruit cup." The communication guide responds by giving the student fruit cup. Next, the student realizes they need a spoon, sees the communication guide holding a spoon and subsequently requests the spoon. The communication guide responds by giving the student the spoon. The student attempts to open fruit cup but is unsuccessful. At this point the student tries to enlist the support of the communication guide by pushing the fruit cup toward them or taking their hand and putting it on top of the fruit cup. This gives the communication guide an opportunity to acknowledge the student's communication by stating, "*I understand* you want help." Then the communication guide models, using hand-over-hand modeling and aided language modeling, "*Your language is* I want help" pointing to symbols on the student's AAC system. Then the guide helps the child open the container. The communication guide comments, pointing to symbols on the student's AAC system, "I like fruit cup." This example illustrates how GLGSP is layered with communication temptations and aided language stimulation.

Table 5–7. Using Communication Temptations to Facilitate Communication

Object	Procedure	Communicative Intent	Language Expectation or Model
Balloon	Blow up a balloon and slowly deflate it. Hand the deflated balloon to the child or hold the deflated balloon to your lips and wait.	Request action Request continuation of preferred activity	Want more Blow it/balloon More blow You do it
Undesired food item or toy	Give the child an undesired food item or object.	Protest	No like (it) No want
Desired food item	Eat a preferred food item in front of student. Make (and model) comments regarding how delicious or enjoyable the food item is.	Request item	I want . . .
Desired food item in closed container	After the child requests a preferred food item, give them the desired food either in the original package (e.g., packet of fruit snacks) or clear container that the student cannot open.	Request action Request assistance	Open it You do it Want help Need help
Ball	Engage the child in a turn-taking activity of rolling a ball back and forth. After several exchanges hold on to the ball and wait for the student to request the ball.	Request action Request object	Want ball Push ball Roll ball
Stuffed animal	Have the stuffed animal greet the child the first time. Repeat this for a second and third time, and do nothing when bringing out the animal the fourth time. These trials should be interspersed when presented.	Greet	Hi Bear

continues

Table 5–7. *continued*

Object	Procedure	Communicative Intent	Language Expectation or Model
Jack in-the-box	Show the student the jack-in-the-box toy and gradually wind the handle until the clown (or other character) jumps out of the box. Observe student's response. At this point the student may request you to put it away (Bye clown, No more) or want to do it again. In the later case, say "Goodbye" and gently return the clown to the box and hand the box to the student. Wait for the student to request assistance.	Request action Greet (or say goodbye) Protest Request object	Want clown No want Go away No more Turn it You turn it I turn it *Lots of communication opportunities with this one
Toy requiring activation	Activate a toy requiring activation (e.g., wind-up toys, toys with buttons or switches that cause an action) and let it run until it turns off, and then hand the deactivated toy to the child.	Request action	Want more Make go You do it I need help
Bubbles	Engage the child in blowing bubbles, return the wand to the container of bubbles, and tightly secure the lid so the student can't open it on their own. Hand the container of bubbles to the student.	Request object Request action	You open You do it Open bubbles More bubbles
Social game (e.g., peek-a-boo)	Engage the student in a social game such peek-a-boo or giving tickles, then abruptly stop the game and wait.	Request action	More play More tickles More go
Swing	Engage in swinging the child, then pause the activity and wait for the student to request more.	Request action Request continuation of preferred activity	You push More swing Make go Go higher

Table 5–7. *continued*

Object	Procedure	Communicative Intent	Language Expectation or Model
Desired drink	Give the student a small amount of their favorite drink in a small cup. Once they finish there will be a need for them to request more. Give them a small amount.	Request item	I want juice Want more More juice
Materials needed for an activity	Give the child some of the materials, but not all of them that are needed to complete the activity such as paper but no glue or scissors, or writing activity but no pencil. Wait for a request. The item needs to be located out of reach of the student; it may or may not be in sight.	Request item Request knowledge	I want . . . I need . . . Where . . .
Necessary item	Provide student with items necessary to complete a task (e.g., glue) in a container they are unable to open independently.	Request action Request assistance	I need help Open it You do it
Car and ramp	Build a car ramp and start with the car at the top and begin a routine of "Ready, Set, Go." After several rounds insert a pause after "Set" waiting for the student to initiate a response.	Request action	Go Make go You go I go Make car go

Source: Ianono, Carter, & Hook, 1998; Prizant & Wetherby, 1985; Wetherby, Cain, Yonclas, & Walker, 1988; Wetherby & Prizant, 1989; Wetherby & Prutting, 1984.

Verbal Behavior

Verbal Behavior is the term used to describe an approach to teaching language based on the principles of applied behavioral analysis (ABA). Verbal Behavior involves strategies that teach children to communicate through operant conditioning. Specifically, a communicative behavior that is delivered by a child that results in a positive response from the environment, such as obtaining a desired food item or receiving a positive reaction from another person, increases the likelihood that behavior will occur again. In a study, Skinner (1957) suggested there was a direct link between communicative acts and behavioral responses of the respondents. In this approach, expression of communication is dependent on the antecedents or the motivation for the behavior and the consequence or the outcome of the communicative behavior (Prelock & Mccauley, 2012). Mands, echoics, and tacts are examples of operant behaviors. Whereas mands dictate generally a physical reinforcer (e.g., cookie in response to "I want cookie"), the other operant communicative behaviors rely on secondary or social reinforcement (e.g., "Nice job!"), which usually comes in the form of social praise or engagement between the communicator and their communication partner.

Mand

A mand is a communicative act that serves to regulate the behavior of another person for the purposes of obtaining a preferred item or action (Prelock & Mccauley, 2012). The antecedent or motivator of the behavior or communicative act elicits a response from the familiar adult or peer, which in turn serves as the consequence or reinforcer.

Tact

A tact is the communicative act of labeling pictures, objects, or actions for the purposes of engaging in joint attention, specifically sharing an experience through commenting (Prelock & Mccauley, 2012). The social interaction that occurs between the child and their communication partner as a result serves as the reinforcer.

Echoic

Echoic is the imitation of another person's communicative act (Prelock & Mccauley, 2012). The ability to imitate another person's communicative behavior—verbal, gestural, and symbol based—is important for overall language learning.

Listener Responding

Listener responding, although not considered a verbal operant, demonstrates the listener's understanding of single word vocabulary and comprehension of directives of varied length and complexity.

As it relates to working with children who are learning to communicate through the use of AAC, it is important to respond to those communicative attempts to increase the likelihood they will occur again. Responding to mands by providing the item or action increases the chances the student will exhibit similar communicative behaviors in the future. Table 5–8 provides examples of how to layer GLGSP and the use of communication temptations to elicit verbal behaviors.

INSTRUCTIONAL CONSIDERATIONS

When students are immersed in a language-rich environment consistent with the language they are trying to learn, and given opportunities to practice using their communication system in meaningful interactions, we create a learning situation that will truly benefit the novice AAC user. We recognize that all students do not learn in the same manner; therefore, we are always customizing our instruction based not only on the needs of the student but in reaction to how they respond. The following are some instructional strategies that have proven effective in supporting students with CCNs benefit from the intervention approach described in this book.

Simplifying Page Set

In Chapter 4 and throughout this chapter, we discuss the need to provide students with access to as many symbols/icons as they can manage. However, having access to too many symbols may, in fact, be overwhelming to the student and affect their ability to accurately select targeted symbols/icons. If this is the case, you might find it effective to "hide" non-targeted cells within the context of a teaching lesson. This is a highly valuable teaching strategy and in fact may be one of the reasons you recommend one AAC application or program over the other. There will be times when having all the icons available to the student is overwhelming and may be hindering their ability to be successful. During specific teaching moments, you may want to only have icons or symbols relevant to the current activity available to the student. In these instances you will want to hide all other icons. Maintain the same location of the targeted symbols and simply hide those the student will not need to have access to during the current activity. When training communication guides during the intervention-planning phase of the intervention process, it will be important to teach them how to quickly hide and unhide icons. It should take a communication guide no more than a couple of minutes (if that) to hide or unhide icons or symbols. It is easier to hide and unhide icons/symbols in some AAC applications and programs compared to others; therefore, if this will be a teaching technique you will be utilizing frequently, you make want to consider this when recommending an AAC application or program. In fact, some AAC systems do not allow you to hide or unhide icons; therefore, you would need to completely reconfigure the student's communication system.

Table 5–8. Verbal Behavior to Facilitate Communication

Verbal Behavior	Motivator (Antecedent)	Communicative Act (Behavior)	Communicative Function (Consequence)	
			Communicative Purpose	Adult/Peer Response
Mand	Feels hungry Sees desired food item or object Communication temptation	"I want (desired item)" "Make go" "Turn on" "No want"	Behavioral Regulation	Uses GLGSP by responding, "I understand" and modeling better or more language if appropriate Gives desired item or responds with requested action
Tact	Sees items of interest Verbal instruction (e.g., "Show me car")	Comments by pointing to or labeling object	Joint Attention	Provides a reinforcing comment (e.g., "That's right!" or "I understand!") Models more language using GLGSP modeling techniques
Echoic	Verbal model Model language on communication system Model language on communication system using GLGSP (e.g., "Your language is . . . 'you open'")	Imitates communication act	Behavioral Regulation Joint Attention Social Interaction	Provides verbal praise (e.g., "I understand you want me to open bubbles"). Responds to communication attempts appropriately

Practice Until Mastery

It is important to support the student until they are capable of executing a skill independently. This requires the adult to balance what the student can currently do and what they can do with modeling, faded prompting, and rehearsal to an independent level. Before you move on to the next step of the activity (e.g., turning the page), you want the student to achieve success. Communication guides are discouraged from "moving on" until the student executes the skills independently. Generally speaking, it should take up to two or three models before the student achieves success but there will be times when you need to stick with it until they are successful. Moving on before the student executes the targeted skill correctly only teaches them that that level of proficiency was sufficient. It is for this reason we must not set our expectation too far above the student's current abilities. It is a constant dance back and forth that requires us to set expectations that are manageable for the student given the right level of support from us. Additionally, always recognize the limitations of hand-over-hand modeling. Students who are the target of the intervention approach described in this book become easily prompt-dependent. Always use the least non-intrusive means to prompt the student. Student will quickly become dependent on hand-over-hand modeling. In fact, many students become passive relying on their communication partners to facilitate them through the communication act.

Lessons and Activities

Select activities and create lessons that are motivating and engaging. Focus less on the end product of an activity and more on the actual process of the activity. Activities that are sensory-based tend to be more motivating for students and keep them engaged longer. For the emergent communicator consider selecting 1 to 3 words or phrases to target per activity or lesson. If you find one aspect or concept of a lesson is unfamiliar, consider including a "break-out lesson." Breakout lessons are small mini-lessons that teach a single concept or vocabulary item to prepare the student for a bigger lesson. Appendix E provides sample activities and lessons that are engaging and motivating, while providing students with CCNs opportunities to use core vocabulary within naturalistic interactions.

PROMOTING GENERALIZATION

Students who are the target of the intervention approach described in this book experience extreme difficulty generalizing new learning to environments that extend beyond the teaching setting. Additionally, they require multiple opportunities to practice these new skills before they become automatic and a part of their repertoire of skills. It is for these reasons the intervention approach described in this book was developed in the manner in which it was. Conventional service delivery models used with this group of students have been provided in one-on-one settings in isolated treatment contexts. Unfortunately, the end result is less significant outcomes for students with CCNs. The American Speech-Language-Hearing Association (2004), endorses a holistic approach to intervention in which individuals who interact with the potential AAC user on a regular basis be involved in the intervention process. This is imperative for the student's success and ultimately generalization of learned skills acquired during the intensive, immersive, socially based intervention. It is for this reason that instructional support staff from the student's regular classroom is included as communication guides. The intensive, immersive, and socially based environment introduced during the intervention is bridged over to the student's classroom, where instructional support staff continue to provide language-rich models, and scaffold opportunities for the student to practice communication skills. The speech-language pathologist or AAC specialist consult with the teacher and instructional support staff to create, implement, and evaluate daily activities within the classroom.

"School-to-Home" Communication Books

Generalization to the home environment is addressed immediately at the onset of the intervention through the use of "School-to-Home" books. These are different than daily communication books. Teachers of students with CCNs frequently use daily communication books, books that go back and forth between the teacher and the parent, as a means to communicate with parents how their child's day went. Contrastively, "School-to-Home" books provide the student with CCNs a medium in which to share with their family what they did at school that day. "School-to-Home" books can take many different forms and usually include comments relative to student's day including what they did or made, what book they read, what they ate, and what was their favorite part of the day. "School-to-Home" books are introduced as part of intervention model and are carried over into the student's classroom. Parents really enjoy these "School-to-Home" books. For many of them, this is the first time their child has ever "told" them about their day.

One way to create a "School-to-Home" book is to create pages for things you want the child to communicate with their family. For example, there may be pages that say, "Today, I ate . . . ," "Today, I made . . . ," Today, I read . . . ." You can even include statements to express emotions. Such "I like to read" or "I no like . . . ." Consistent with the principles of the intervention approach discussed in this book are that each word should be paired with a symbol compatible with the student's AAC language. It is suggested that pages be laminated and Velcro used to attach symbols to reflect the day's events and activities. At the end of each day, time should be set aside to review the student's "School-to-Home" communication book and make sure it reflects the student's day. Feel free to be creative in how you develop your student's "School-to-Home." It should reflect his or her needs and abilities and be easily implemented by classroom staff and parents. Figure 5–1 provides a sample letter you can send home with parents to explain the purpose of the "School-to-Home" and how to use it.

School to Home Books

Dear Parents,

We are excited to work with your child this new school year! Our goal is to focus on teaching your child to communicate in multiple environments using core and fringe vocabulary words. Core vocabulary are words that can be used across a variety of environments, (I, my, is, get, do, want). Fringe words are those words that are specific to a certain environment or activity (glue, red, bubbles, goldfish). Your child is bringing home their "School-to-Home" book. The purpose of the "School to Home" book is to give your child an opportunity to share with you a little about their day. For example, what they ate, what they made, and what their favorite activity was. We suggest you create a routine every day to ask your child about their day. Below is a script of the type of language you can use to elicit communication with your child:

"Hi _____, what did you do at school today? or, Tell me about your day" "You read a book? Your language is, "I read a book" (pointing to symbols with their finger to "read" the symbols). "Wow, it sounds like you had a great day. What was the favorite thing you did today?" Have your child flip through and find their favorite activity. They can point to the symbols and "read" it to you. If they made a craft, take that time to pull it out of their backpack and point to different parts and talk about the colors, materials used, what it does, and ask simple yes/no questions to elicit a response.

It is important that your child bring their "School to Home" book with them to school each day so that the day's activities can be recorded and sent back home.

We look forward to working with your child and having a fantastic school year! If you have any questions, please feel free to call the school or send a note with them.

Sincerely,

_____

Figure 5–1. A sample letter you can send home with parents to explain the purpose of the "School-to-Home" and how to use it.

MOVING STUDENT TOWARD
COMMUNICATIVE COMPETENCE

It cannot be emphasized enough that AAC-based interventions are not a single technique but a constant layering of techniques and strategies. If we want to ensure a student's success, we make sure they are engaged in the process and experience the benefits of communication. Communication should be a positive experience so we can show students what they can accomplish through communication.

REFERENCES

American Speech-Language-Hearing Association. (2004). *Roles and responsibilities of speech-language pathologists with respect to augmentative and alternative communication* [Technical report]. Available from http://www.asha.org/policy

Beck, A., Stoner, J. B., & Dennis, M. L. (2009). An investigation of aided language stimulation: Does it increase AAC use with adults with developmental disabilities and complex communication needs? *Augmentative and Alternative Communication, 25*(1), 42–54.

Beukelman, D.R., & Mirenda, P. (2013). *Augmentative and alternative communication: Supporting children and adults with complex communication needs* (4th ed.). Baltimore, MD: Paul Brookes.

Binger, C., Berens, J., Kent-Walsh, J., & Taylor, S. (2008). The effect of aided AAC interventions on AAC use, speech, and symbol gestures. *Seminars in Speech and Language 29*(2), 101–111.

Binger, C., & Light, J. (2007). The effect of aided AAC modeling on the expression of multi-symbol messages by preschoolers who use AAC. *Augmentative and Alternative Communication, 23*(1), 30–43.

Binger, C., Maguire-Marshall, M., & Kent-Walsh, J. (2011). Using aided models, recasts, and contrastive targets to teach grammatical morphemes to children who use AAC. *Journal of Speech, Language, and Hearing Research, 54*, 160–176.

Bruno, J., & Trembath, D. (2006). Use of aided language stimulation to improve syntactic performance during a weeklong intervention program. *Augmentative and Alternative Communication, 22*(4), 300–313.

Cafiero, J. (1998). Communication power for individuals with autism. *Focus on Autism and Other Developmental Disabilities, 13*, 113–121.

Cirrin, F. M., Schooling, T. L., Nelson, N. W., Diehl, S. F., Flynn, P., Staskowski, M., . . . Adamczyk, D. F. (2010). Effects of different service delivery models on communication outcomes for elementary school-age children. *Language, Speech, and Hearing Services in Schools, 41*,233–264.

Dada, S., & Alant, E. (2009). The effect of aided language stimulation on vocabulary acquisition in children with little or no functional speech. *American Journal of Speech-Language Pathology, 18*, 50–64.

Dodd, J. L. (2011). Creating early literacy opportunities for children with complex communication needs. In M. F. Shaughnessy & K. Kleyn (Eds.), *Handbook of early childhood education*. Hauppauge, NY: Nova Science.

Drager, K. R., Postal, V. J., Carrolus, L., Castellano, M., Gagliano, C., & Glynn, J. (2006). The effect of aided language modeling on symbol comprehension and production in 2 preschoolers with autism. *American Journal of Speech-Language Pathology, 15*(2), 112–125. http://dx.doi.org/10.1044/1058-0360(2006/012)

Goossens', C. (1989). Aided communication intervention before assessment: A case study of a child with cerebral palsy. *AAC Augmentative and Alternative Communication, 5,* 14–26.

Harris, M. D., & Reichle, J. (2004). The impact of aided language stimulation on symbol comprehension and production in children with moderate cognitive disabilities. *American Journal of Speech-Language Pathology, 13,* 155–167.

Holdaway, D. (1979). *The foundations of learning.* New York, NY: Scholastic.

Ianono, T., Carter, M., & Hook, J. (1998). Identification of intentional communication in students with severe and multiple disabilities. *Augmentative and Alternative Communication, 14,* 102–113

Jonsson, A., Kristoffersson, L., Ferm, U., & Thunberg, G. (2011). The ComAlong communication boards: Parents' use and experiences of aided language stimulation. *Augmentative and Alternative Communication, 27*(2), 103–116. http://dx.doi.org/10.3109/07434618.2011.580780

Justice, L. M., & Pence, K. L. (2005). *Scaffolding with storybooks: A guide for enhancing young children's language and literacy achievement.* Newark, DE: International Reading Association.

Kent-Walsh, J., & Mcnaughton, D. (2005). Communication partner instruction in AAC: Present practices and future directions. *Augmentative and Alternative Communication, 21*(3), 195–204. http://dx.doi.org/10.1080/07434610400006646

Lund, S. K., & Light, J. (2003). The effectiveness of grammar instruction for individuals who use augmentative and alternative communicative systems: A preliminary study. *Journal of Speech, Language, and Hearing Research, 46,* 1110–1123.

Moore, B. J., & Montgomery, J. K. (2017). *Speech language pathologists in public schools: Making a difference for America's children* (3rd ed.). Austin, TX: Pro-Ed.

Nigam, R., Schlosser, R., & Lloyd, L. (2006). Concomitant use of the matrix strategy and the mand-model procedure in teaching graphic symbol combinations. *Augmentative and Alternative Communication, 22,* 160–177.

Paul, R., & Norbury, C. F. (2012). *Language disorders from infancy through adolescence: Listening, speaking, reading, writing, and communicating* (4th ed.). St. Louis, MO: Elsevier Mosby.

Prelock, P. A., & McCauley, R. J. (2012). *Treatment of autism spectrum disorders: Evidence-based instruction for communication and social interactions.* Baltimore, MD: Paul H. Brookes.

Prizant, B., & Wetherby, A. (1985). Intentional communicative behavior of children with autism: Theoretical and practice issues. *Australian Journal of Human Communication Disorders, 13,* 21–59.

Romski, M. A., & Sevcik, R. A. (1996). *Breaking the speech barrier: Language development through augmented means.* York, PA: Brookes.

Romski, M. A., & Sevcik, R. A. (2003). Augmented input: Enhancing communication development. In J. Light, D. Beukelman, & J. Reichle (Eds.), *Communicative competence for individuals who use AAC* (pp. 147–162). Baltimore, MD: Paul H. Brookes.

Romski, M. A., Sevcik, R. A., & Adamson, L. B. (1999). Communication patterns of youth with mental retardation with and without their speech-output communication devices. *American Journal On Mental Retardation, 104*(3), 249–259.

Scherer, N., & Olswang, L. (1984). Role of mothers' expansions in stimulating language production. *Journal of Speech and Hearing Research, 27,* 387–396.

Senner, J. E. (2008, July 23). *Partner augmented input* [Instructional video]. Retrieved from http://www.dynavoxtech.com/implementation-toolkit/details.aspx?id=261

Skatvoid, S. K. (1976). The general-language general-speech pattern (GLGSP). *Language, Speech, and Hearing Services in Schools, 7,* 190–196.

Skinner, B. F. (1957). *Verbal behavior.* Upper Saddle River, NJ: Prentice-Hall.

Warren, S. F., Fey, M. E., & Yoder, P. J. (2007). Differential treatment intensity research: A missing to creating optimally effective communication interventions. *Mental Retardation and Developmental Disabilities Research Reviews, 13*(1), 70–77.

Wetherby, A. M., Cain, D. H., Yonclas, D. G., & Walker, V. G. (1988). Analysis of intentional communication of normal children from the pre-linguistic to the multiword stage. *Journal of Speech and Hearing Research, 31,* 240–252.

Wetherby, A. M., & Prizant, B. M. (1989). The expression of communicative intent: Assessment guidelines. *Seminars in Speech and Language, 10*(1), 77–91.

Wetherby, A. M., & Prutting, C. A. (1984). Profiles of communicative and cognitive abilities in autistic children. *Journal of Speech and Hearing Research, 27,* 364–377.

Wilkinson, K. M., Romski, M. A., & Sevcik, R. A. (1994). Emergence of visual-graphic symbol combinations by youth with moderate or severe mental retardation. *Journal of Speech and Hearing Research, 37*(4), 883–895.

Yaden, D. B. (1989). Understanding stories through repeated read-alouds: How many does it take? *The Reading Teacher, 41,* 556–561.

CHAPTER 6

Progress Monitoring

Progress monitoring, as it relates to students with disabilities, is the scientific practice of assessing a student's progress and evaluating the effectiveness of an intervention. Monitoring a student's progress is good clinical practice and a mandate under federal law. The Individuals with Disabilities Education Act (IDEA) (2004) stipulates that a student's individualized education program (IEP) include "a statement of the student's present levels of academic achievement and functional performance . . . [and] a statement of measurable annual goals" (34 CFR 300.320). Progress monitoring, as a practice, gives intervention teams the performance data necessary to make informed instructional decisions. From an annual perspective, progress monitoring details what the student has learned and what gaps continue to exist. In addition to evaluating a student's long-term progress, it is necessary to monitor their short-term response as well. This allows the team to appraise the student's response to the intervention so modifications and adjustments can be made to get the most out of the student's long-term response to the intervention itself. While frequently assessing a student's response has application to a wide range of interventions, it has particular relevance to students who are learning to use augmentative and alternative communication (AAC). An AAC-based intervention does not follow a formulaic course with predictive next steps. Rather, it is a fluid process of adaptations in reaction to the student's response to the intervention. Therefore, it is important to periodically evaluate how a student is responding to a particular intervention so that alterations can be made to boost the student's progression. AAC intervention requires constant customization.

Monitoring a student's progress is a necessary component of the intervention presented in this book. Informed decisions, which serve as the basis for developing, implementing, and modifying a well-focused intervention plan, are driven by data. Data-based decision making entails the gathering of objective data so that informed decisions are made. Objective data allow intervention teams to evaluate, without bias, a student's true response to an intervention. When intervention teams use systematic progress monitoring techniques to track a student's response, they are able to identify what is working for the student and what adjustments need to be made to strengthen the instructional program, and ultimately help their student achieve better results.

Documenting progress in students with complex communication needs (CCNs) can be difficult. Students with CCNs often progress at a slower rate and their achievement of well-intentioned targets is often thwarted from the beginning by the intervention itself or the limitations of their communication system. As discussed in Chapter 1, many interventions typically used with this population fall short in facilitating key components of communication (e.g., *social competence*). Additionally, many children who benefit from AAC-based interventions often demonstrate small incremental changes that may go undetected if the sensitivity of the assessment measure is not discreet enough. In fact, current progress monitoring techniques may fail to document the progress these students are making. Measuring a student's response to an intervention is not only a legal mandate under federal law (IDEA) and necessary in documenting progress towards IEP goals, but important in developing and implementing an evidenced-based instructional program.

Federal law (IDEA, 2004) mandates intervention teams monitor treatment effectiveness. Interventionists often find it difficult to document progress in students who are the target of the intervention described in this book. It is can be perceived that the student is not making progress when in fact they are. How the goals were written may not be effective in demonstrating the progress many of these students are capable of making. Students with CCNs, such as those diagnosed with severe forms of autism or other equally communicatively and socially impairing disorders, progress at a slow rate, which can be difficult to quantify. Therefore, operative progress monitoring for this population is reliant on two processes: (a) a measure that is sensitive enough to document change and (b) an intervention that is effective in inducing change.

Determining the effectiveness (or ineffectiveness) of the intervention, which guides teams in making informed decisions regarding necessary modifications required to progress the child toward the desired outcomes, is a necessary component of the intervention process. There is nothing more discouraging for both parents and practitioners than attending an IEP meeting annually only to report that goals are continually "not met." Goals repeatedly reported as "not met" lead parents to lose faith in the team's ability to progress their child to the next level.

MONITORING PROGRESS

The argument has been made regarding the importance (and federally mandated obligation) of monitoring a student's response to an intervention. Now it is time to examine how progress monitoring can be accomplished both efficiently and effectively with students who are learning to use an AAC system. It is important that progress monitoring be efficient. If the manner in which data are gathered is laborious or time consuming, it is less likely to be conducted on a regular basis, which will negatively impact a student's progress. Implementing an AAC-based intervention is a fluid process that requires constant fine-tuning as the student's needs change from week to week, day to day, subject to subject, and even class to class. Therefore, if the method of monitoring the student's progress is efficient, it will be conducted on a regular basis, giving the team access to the data needed to make adaptations that will positively impact the student's outcome. Effective goes hand-in-hand with efficiency. Specific, detailed data will guide you in making those adaptations that will have the greatest impact on moving your student forward toward their goals. Data-driven decisions have a direct impact on students' successes.

The customary way to evaluate a student's progress to a particular intervention is to develop goals and measure his or her progress towards those goals. The challenge is how to write goals for students who are using AAC —not only as a means to communicate, but as a means to learn how to communicate (Dodd & Gorey, 2014). While goal writing for students who use AAC share many commonalities to those written for verbal children, there are some distinct differences (e.g., application of technology, AAC-related skills) that must be considered, including the application of technology and proficiency in AAC-related skills.

As previously stated, the overreaching goal and philosophical foundation of the intervention described in this book is to facilitate the emergence of competent communicators. Targeting only one area (e.g., linguistic) fails to address the other necessary components of AAC communication (e.g., socialization, strategies to repair communicative breakdown, etc.). Effective AAC interventions target all four competency areas (Light, 1989; Light & McNaughton, 2014). Keep in mind that this framework will be especially helpful when creating goals for AAC users. Goal development, as it relates to AAC use, is a cyclical process that must be constantly revisited. Goal development begins with establishing a student's present level of performances (PLOPs) in each of the four competency areas. From that point, intervention needs are identified and measurable, and relevant goals are developed. Progress towards these goals is continually monitored as the student's abilities and needs change, and goals are again adjusted. This is a continual process that must be revisited on a regular basis for consistent progress to occur.

WRITING PRESENT LEVELS OF PERFORMANCE (PLOPS)

The purpose of writing present levels of performance (PLOPs) is to establish a baseline of skills and to describe the unique needs of the child from which goals can be developed and addressed through intervention. The term "performance" is used to describe what the child can do in objective, measurable terms, incorporating information from a variety of resources. PLOPs are generally written in two areas: academic skills (also referred to as present levels of educational performance) and functional skills. Functional skills refer to those abilities that are necessary for participation in routine activities of daily living, including self-help skills (e.g., toileting, dressing), social skills, communication, behavior, and mobility. PLOPs can be determined using standardized tests, but are also determined through data collected by observing the student throughout his/her day, receiving input from the parent and teacher, and reviewing performance on previous goals. PLOPs are based on all information and data collected about the child, and typically includes both quantitative and qualitative forms of information. Quantitative data, performance data reported in numerical form (e.g., 4 out of 5 times, with 80% accuracy), are considered the more objective, measurable means of the two forms with regard to reporting performance levels. However, it is often necessary and appropriate to include qualitative forms of information as well to describe behavior or information that cannot be easily measured using more traditional quantitative means The limitation of qualitative data is that it is generally gathered through observation based on interpretative knowledge, which can be problematic, as our observations can be influenced by what we want to see.

With respect to communication, it is important to write PLOPs in each of the four competency areas (i.e., linguistic, operational, social, and strategic). Begin by describing the student's performance in a broad sense and then becoming more specific. Avoid describing what the student cannot do (e.g., Johnny does not use verbal language to communicate), instead focusing on the abilities of the student (e.g., Johnny uses the manual sign "more" to indicate continuation of a preferred activity). The following general guidelines and suggestions review writing PLOPs in each of the four competency areas. This is by no means an exclusive list, but rather some general thoughts of the types of information that could be included.

◆ PLOPs in the area of *linguistic competence* can report how many symbols/phrases the student uses, noting the number of fringe versus core words (e.g., "Trevor consistently uses the 'I want' symbol paired with preferred food items." or "Chuck demonstrates understanding and use of 10 core vocabulary words and 8 fringe words."). A student may seem to present with a high number of symbol knowledge, but if that lexicon is predominately composed of fringe words, they may struggle to use their communication system for purposes other than requesting "things." It is also important to denote how many symbols the student is sequencing to compose a message, and the types of sentence structures they are constructing (e.g., action + object, actor + action + object). How many symbols are they using on a regular basis to construct their messages? Are they constructing sentences with "I want" as a single picture icon, or as separate icons (i.e., "I" + "want")? Answering these key questions provides a comprehensive description of the student's linguistic competence related to their AAC use.

> A sample PLOP for linguistic competence: *Sam's AAC vocabulary consists of two core vocabulary words and eight fringe words. Sam demonstrates understanding and use of the core vocabulary words "want" and "more" that he pairs with preferred food items (i.e., cookies, chips, juice, fish-crackers,) and activities (i.e., swing, ball, puzzle).*

◆ PLOPs in the area of *operational competence* can describe how well the student uses his or her device, and includes, statements regarding their access abilities (e.g., direct access, scanning), the number of cells on a page, and whether or not they are using a static or dynamic display configuration. This area also describes their navigational skills with respect to turning on/off their device, turning up/down the volume, deleting a message, and activating a message after composing it. It also describes their ability to navigate through their AAC system to a desired item or activity-specific page and their ability to return to the home page.

> Sample PLOPs for operational competence: *Kaitlin turns on/off her AAC system (i.e., iPad mini programmed with the Proloquo2Go app) when given the verbal prompt, "Use your words." She uses direct selection to access cells from a field of 32 icons. She navigates to folders containing preferred food items (i.e., snack) and classroom reinforcers. She needs hand-over-hand prompting to activate the message bar after constructing a three-symbol message and to return to her home page.*

◆ PLOPs in the area of *social competence* describe those skills related to the social use of language. It is important to describe the purposes for which the student uses his or her communication system (e.g., "Samantha uses 1 to 2 symbol messages to request preferred food items during snack and desired reinforces upon completion of a non-preferred activity."). Individuals who use AAC are more likely to assume the discourse role of a responder; therefore, it is important to note the student's rate of initiations in comparison to responses.

> Sample PLOPs for social competence: *Charlie responds to question prompts (e.g., "What do you want?"). Ninety percent of Charlie's communicative messages are responses. Charlie occasionally initiates communication for highly preferred food items.*

◆ PLOPs in the area of *strategic competence* incorporate those skills an AAC user employs to compensate for the shortcomings of their AAC system. AAC systems give students access to a finite number of words, and often the words they can access must serve multiple functions. Additionally, many of the students who are considered candidates for this intervention approach are often passive in their communication attempts. These students frequently need to learn how to be persistent in conveying messages. Does the student recognize when there was a failed communication attempt? What strategies do they apply when there is a failed communication attempt (e.g., repeat the message, rephrase the message)? Also within this area of competency, it is important to describe the student's use of aberrant, socially unacceptable behaviors to communicate frustration, need for assistance, or, better yet, to request a break.

> Sample PLOPs for strategic competence: *Given a non-preferred activity, Chuck will scream and elope to escape from the activity. If his attempts are intentionally or non-intentionally ignored, he will either respond by sitting quietly, walking away to engage in an alternative activity of interest, or respond by throwing himself on the floor. His response is directly influenced by his overall motivation of his request.*

As previously mentioned, it is best practice to write PLOPs by stating what the child *can do*. Although this may seem obvious, avoid stating what they can do by stating what they cannot do. For example instead of reporting, *Vince does not recognize when there is a failed communication attempt,* write, *In response to a failed communication attempt Vince will wait until he is prompted to repeat the message (e.g., "What do you want?")* Instead of reporting, *Charlie does not currently use an AAC system,* describe his current means of communicating his wants and needs. For example, *Charlie uses vocalizations and varied pitch to indicate basic wants.*

IDENTIFYING AREA OF NEEDS AND DEVELOPING GOALS

Identifying intervention targets for a student takes into consideration their PLOPs, combined with expectations of the environment. What types of communication skills does the student need to exhibit in order to be an active participant in their environment? What skills need to be established to assist them in achieving a greater level of participation? As we know, sometimes there are several skills that need to be acquired prior to reaching the long-term goal. Knowing the student's current level of functioning relative to desired outcome enables teams to begin to develop skills towards achievement of long-term goals. The following are lists of potential target skills per competency area appropriate to students who are developing their communication, regardless of their means of communication.

Potential intervention targets related to *linguistic competence*:

- ◆ Increase symbol knowledge and use
- ◆ Increase the average number of symbols sequenced to compose a message
- ◆ Expand types of sentence constructions (e.g., actor-action-object)

Potential intervention targets related to *social competence*:

- ◆ Increase rate of initiation for preferred and non-preferred activities
- ◆ Increase rate of communicative acts
- ◆ Increase social responsiveness
- ◆ Expand range of purposes for communication

Potential intervention targets related to *operational competence*:

- ◆ Navigate back to home page
- ◆ Activate message bar
- ◆ Turn system on/off
- ◆ Transition AAC system from one activity to the next
- ◆ Locate activity specific pages/folders

Potential intervention targets related to *strategic competence*:

- ◆ Develop a means to indicate a need for assistance, an activity is too hard, he/she does not like the activity
- ◆ Recognize a failed communication attempt
- ◆ Repair a communication breakdown
- ◆ Use a single term for multiple functions

Once intervention needs are identified it is important to develop goals that are both measurable and achievable.

WRITING SMART GOALS

Our discussion on writing goals for students with CCN begins with reviewing best practices for writing goals. When it comes to writing goals for students with complex communication needs we want to make sure we are being S.M.A.R.T. about it! The field of special education has adopted the concept of SMART goal writing, which was originally introduced in 1981 by George

Doran in the November, 1981 issue of the *Management Review,* to writing IEP goals. SMART is a mnemonic acronym that "spells out" a criteria/guideline for developing specific, measurable, attainable, realistic, timely (tangible) goals. SMART goal writing is considered one of the most effective tools used by high achievers and is instituted by large business owners, small business entrepreneurs, and even individuals seeking a healthier life style. A well-written SMART goal explicitly states what an individual will do and under what condition, how accomplishment of that goal will be determined, and identifies an expected date of accomplishment.

SMART Goals:	S-Specific
	M-Measurable
	A-Attainable
	R-Realistic
	T-Timely

In order to understand the application of SMART goal writing to AAC, let's begin by defining the features of SMART goals and how they relate to AAC.

Specific: SMART Goals Are Specific

Specific goals include clear descriptions of the desired outcome. Focused goals specify the intended direction of a targeted behavior (i.e., increase, decrease, maintain), how progress will be measured, under what condition progress will be measured, and the level of attainment (i.e., to age level, without assistance, with one adult prompt, etc.). Goals that are specifically written are easier to measure and have a greater chance of being accomplished than general goals. Non-specific goals describe desired outcomes in a general sense (e.g., "communicate" or "participate in classroom activities") whereas specific goals state specific skills a student is expected to achieve (e.g., use 10 core vocabulary words). Specific goals answer six specific questions so that it is clear to everyone what the targeted outcome will be. The following provides examples of these questions as they relate to AAC:

Who is involved? Charlie

What is the desired outcome? Use two symbol messages consisting of core and fringe vocabulary words

Where will this behavior occur? In the classroom

When *will this behavior be achieved by?* By January 19, 2017

Which *conditions?* Given a communication opportunity

Why *is this behavior important/necessary?* To request preferred food items and objects

Measurable

Writing goals that are measurable can be tricky. In general, goals are written in terms of accuracy of targeted behavior (e.g., with 80% accuracy) or frequency of occurrence (e.g., four out of five times). When identifying the criteria, it is important your measurement is easily interpreted and collected. This is the tricky part. For example, if you want to increase social interaction writing a goal to "greet peers in 80% of opportunities" might be confusing because the definition of an "opportunity" is not clearly defined and may be interpreted differently by different people. The goal could be changed to "greet peers within 30 seconds of entering a new environment" to make it more easily measurable. It is also important to write goals a student can achieve inde-pendently at a high rate of accuracy (e.g., 80 to 90% accuracy). It is important to strive to not only write measurable goals, but goals a student can execute independently (to the maximum extent possible) with a high rate of accuracy. Remember, if the student exceeds expectations and meets their goal early, you should add a new goal to continue the progress they have already achieved.

Achievable

While a goal should push an individual to achieve to their highest level, a goal should not be unsurmountable either. As well as, it is important to avoid writing goals that underestimate a student's potential. It is somewhat of a balancing act between writing goals that are challenging, yet achievable. If a student is new to you, it may be challenging at first to fully recognize or understand their rate of learning. It is best practice to write a goal you antici-pate a student can achieve in the designated time period (e.g., annually) based on your own clinical judgment and related expertise.

Relevant

Meaningful goals can help AAC users, especially new AAC users, stay engaged in the learning process. Goals that focus on drill rather than more functional activities may not seem as relevant to an AAC user and, as a result, may not be reached as quickly. Although it is common practice to select goals from sets of pre-established written communication goals, it is important to modify and individualize goals to address the unique needs and disability of a particular student, taking into consideration the communication demands of their environment.

Time Limited: Goals Need to Have an Ending Point

Begin by considering the baseline and present levels of the student, and then decide what they can accomplish within a year. Annual goals should be monitored regular intervals to ensure the student is progressing as would be expected.

SMART GOALS APPLIED TO IEP GOALS

SMART IEP goals are specific, measureable, achievable, relevant, and timely, leaving little room for interpretation. The SMART IEP goals state the achiever's name, what they will achieve under what condition, when this outcome will be achieved by, and how achievement will be determined and measured. Figure 6–1 illustrates the components of SMART IEP goals.

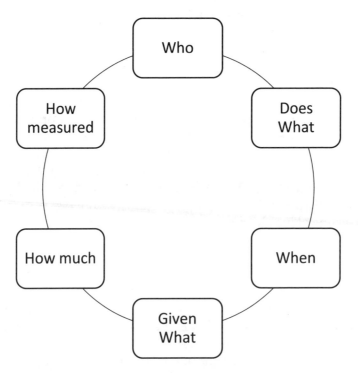

Figure 6–1. Components of SMART IEP Goals.

Table 6–1. Action Words Used To Describe Target Behaviors

Use	Construct	Formulate	Respond	Initiate
Demonstrate	Request	Comment	Ask	Interact
Greet	Select	Participate	Provide	Compose
Activate	Navigate	Maintain	Terminate	Engage
Recognize	Access	Locate		

SMART IEP goals describe the desired behavior that will be achieved in action terms. The following describes each component of the IEP goal formula and provides an example of how it may be written.

Who: The student—*Elizabeth*

Given What: Under what condition desired behavior will occur— *Given a shared reading activity and verbal prompt to use her device*

Does What: Observable behavior described in action terms (see Table 6–1 for a list of action words appropriate for describing target behavior in action terms)—*Construct two- to three-symbol messages consisting of at least one core and one fringe word to answer questions*

When: Due date—*By April 5, 2017*

How Much: Level of accomplishment—*On four out of five opportunities*

How Measured: *As measured by speech-language pathologist observation and data*

Here is an example of a SMART IEP goal written using this formula:

By 3/15/2017 (WHEN), *given a shared reading activity and verbal prompt to use her device* (GIVEN WHAT), *Elizabeth* (WHO) *will construct two- to three-symbol messages consisting of at least one core word and one fringe word to answer teacher questions* (DO WHAT) *five times within a story* (HOW MUCH).

SAMPLE GOALS

As we strive to promote a student towards achievement of communicative competence we are reminded that communicative competence is achieved when the individual exhibits proficiency across the four competency areas. Therefore, no less than one goal should be written in each of the four competency areas. The following sample goals provide examples of how goals can be developed to target a wide range of skills in the areas of linguistic competence, operational competence, social competence and strategic competence. Personalize goals referring to the student by name, in these examples replacing STUDENT with the child's actual name. The goals listed here are geared toward individuals who are often described as "beginning communicators" or "emergent communicators."

Linguistic Goals

These goals facilitate not only the receptive and expressive language skills of the student's native language(s) but also the knowledge of the linguistic code unique to their AAC system (e.g., picture symbols, line drawings, real photos, words) (Light, 1989; Light & McNaughton, 2014).

- Given a field of 12 icons, STUDENT will select a single symbol to request preferred objects and activities.
- Given a field of 30 icons, STUDENT will construct two-symbol messages to request preferred food items.
- Given a field of 16 icons, STUDENT will participate in a structured activity using two-symbol phrases.
- Given a field of 30 icons, STUDENT will construct two- to three-symbol messages consisting of at least one core word and one fringe word.
- Posed a verbal question, STUDENT will provide a reliable yes/no response.
- Given access to a communication system consisting of 32 picture icons/symbols/cells, STUDENT will demonstrate understanding and use of 16 core vocabulary words.
- Given communication opportunities. STUDENT will consistently use three-symbol messages to communicate and participate.
- Given a shared reading activity, STUDENT will independently respond to teacher directed questions (e.g., "Where is the cat?") using two- to-three-symbol messages no less than five times within an activity.
- Given a "where" question prompt, STUDENT will respond using core vocabulary (e.g., in there, on it, there, here, it there, not here) with 80% accuracy.
- Given a structured activity, STUDENT will use messages on average three symbols in length to participate in classroom activities.
- Given an adult lead activity, STUDENT will use the prepositions "in" and "on" to indicate location.
- Given a field of preferred and non-referred objects and activities, STUDENT will communicate a preference no less that two times per activity.

◆ STUDENT will use a minimum of three different two-symbol language constructions (e.g., actor-action, action-object, negation, questions) to participate in classroom activities (Tables 6–2, 6–3, and 6–4 list potential language construction).

Operational Goals

Encompass goals that target the technical skills needed for effective and efficient operation of the student's AAC system (Light, 1989; Light & McNaughton, 2014). There are other more advanced operational goals (e.g.,

Table 6–2. Single Symbol Language Constructions

Actors	Actions	Objects	Prepositions	Negation	Locatives	Misc.
I	Want	It	In	Not/don't	Here	More
You	Stop	That	On		There	All done
	Help		Off			
	Eat					
	Drink					
	Like					

Table 6–3. Two-Symbol Language Constructions

Actor-Action	Action-Object	Action-Location	Object-Action	Location-Object
I want	Eat it	Put there	It go	In there/cup
You go	Turn it/page	Put on		
I help	Push it/ball			
	Get that			
	Open juice			

Action-Location	Possession	Questions	Negation
Put in	My turn	What that?	Not here
Put on	Your turn	What go?	No more
			No want

Table 6–4. Three-Symbol Message Constructions

Sentence Construction	Examples	
Actor-Action-Object	I want that/juice	You stop it
	You get it	I do it
	I like it	You do it
	You open it	I got it
Action-Object-Location	Put it on	Push it here
Actor-Object-Location	You go there	You put on
Negation	I don't like	Don't do that
	No more go	

programming one's own device) but the goals listed here address the operational skills relevant to an emergent or beginning communicator.

◆ Given a communication opportunity, STUDENT will demonstrate the ability to accurately locate and access a picture symbol on his/her device.

◆ STUDENT will demonstrate use of at least X navigational tools (on, off, clear, go back, delete).

◆ Given a communication opportunity, STUDENT will compose a message and then activate the message bar.

◆ Given a structured activity, STUDENT will correctly select a category folder to navigate to activity-related symbols for a minimum of three classroom/school-based activities.

◆ STUDENT will navigate through X levels to locate symbols of preferred items and activities.

◆ Given an activity or subject, STUDENT will navigate to the related activity/subject specific page.

◆ Given a communication opportunity, STUDENT will use his/her index finger to select appropriate symbol on device.

◆ Given a communication opportunity, STUDENT will activate his/her communication device and select the appropriate communication app.

◆ Given access to a communication system consisting of 32 picture icons/symbols/cells (and a key guard), STUDENT will use direct select (e.g., index finger) to activate intended cells on four out of five opportunities.

◆ STUDENT will independently transfer his/her communication device to various locations/activities throughout his/her school day.

◆ STUDENT will navigate to the home page.

◆ STUDENT will adjust the volume to accommodate the noise level of the current environment.
◆ Given a dynamic screen AAC device or app, STUDENT will navigate from the core language screen to at least four other screens.

Social Goals

Target the skills of social interactions such as initiating, maintaining, developing, and terminating communication interactions (Light, 1989; Light & McNaughton, 2014). Social goals facilitate the pragmatic use of communication for an expanding range of purposes such as labeling objects, commenting, requesting and sharing information, expressing feelings, and directing the actions of others. Refer to Table 3–4 for a comprehensive list of communicative functions including examples relevant to early communicators.

◆ Given a communication opportunity, STUDENT will use their communication device to direct the behavior of another person.
◆ Given a communication opportunity, STUDENT will use their communication device to share information with another person/familiar adult/peer.
◆ Given a social interaction opportunity with peers, STUDENT will use their AAC system to comment on a shared activity.
◆ Given a field of X icons, STUDENT will ask a communication partner a question related to a shared activity.
◆ Given a field of X icons, STUDENT will use a one-symbol message on device to request, reject, greet others, or comment.
◆ STUDENT will spontaneously use their communication system to request preferred objects or activities no less than 10 times during a 2-hour period.
◆ Upon observing an item of interest, STUDENT will comment about the object (e.g., label the object, "it there," "look") for the purpose of establishing shared attention no less than five times within their regular school day.
◆ STUDENT will greet at least one peer or familiar adult within one minute of entering a new environment no less than five times within their regular school day.
◆ Given a communication opportunity, STUDENT will increase his/her initiative responses by 50%.
◆ STUDENT will use their AAC system to ask partner-focused questions (e.g., What do you like? You like? Where go?) to one adult and one peer.
◆ STUDENT will use their AAC system to invite a peer to play (e.g., come play).

- Given their AAC system, STUDENT will interact with a peer and take three to four conversational turns related to the current activity or topic.
- STUDENT will use their AAC system to greet or say goodbye to a peer when they enter or leave an environment at least 10 times per day.
- STUDENT will use their AAC system to label objects within his/her immediate environment no less than 10 times per day.

Strategic Goals

Teach the compensatory strategies necessary to compensate for the limitations associated with using an AAC system (Light, 1989; Light & McNaughton, 2014).

- Given a communication breakdown, STUDENT will demonstrate persistence by repeating the intended message on their device when their communication partner does not respond.
- Given a communication breakdown, STUDENT will demonstrate persistence by gesturing (e.g., waving, tapping) to gain the attention of their communication partner.
- Given a communication breakdown, STUDENT will recognize the need to repeat and/or alter the original message when their communication attempt is misunderstood, missed or ignored.
- Given a communication opportunity, STUDENT will use at least three different core vocabulary words for a minimum of two different purposes each (e.g., LIKE—I like it, like you; TURN—I turn it, my turn).
- Given a communication opportunity when their device is out of reach, STUDENT will appropriately request/obtain their device.
- Given a frustrating situation, STUDENT will request appropriate supports (e.g., request a break, request assistance).

MONITORING A STUDENT'S RESPONSE TO INTERVENTION

Monitoring a student's response to an intervention should not be a complicated process given you have a clear plan of what types of data you want to gather, how that data will be recorded, and how it will be analyzed, reported, and/or used. Data should be collected on a daily basis and will vary depending on your intended use for that information. There are times when data collected are used to evaluate a student's acquisition of a specific skill. Other times data are collected to evaluate the effectiveness of the intervention or to guide changes or modifications necessary to ensure continued progression of skills. Sometimes data have to be collected to report on present levels of performance. The type and extent of data collected will vary depending on intended purpose of the information collected. Data are collected on a daily basis to evaluate how a student is progressing towards long-term goals (e.g., upon completion of the two-week intervention, within a year), short-term objectives (e.g., activity, session, week, monthly, reporting period), and session/daily targets.

Annual Goals

Measurable annual goals, a mandate under federal law (IDEA, 2004), are statements that describe what a student is expected to accomplish within a 12-month period in the student's educational program. The term "goal" will be used throughout this book to refer to any desired outcome following a specified period of intervention.

Short-Term and Benchmark Objectives

The terms "short-term objectives" and "benchmark objectives" are sometimes mistakenly used synonymously. Collectively, they refer to the "measurable, intermediate steps that enable families, students, and educators to monitor progress during the year, and, if appropriate, to revise the IEP consistent with the child's instructional needs" (Bateman & Linden, 1998, p. 43). The term *benchmark* is applicable when describing a change in the percentage or the accuracy of the behavior that is the end result of the annual goal. When the skills leading to the annual goal are different or are an intermediary step, the term *short-term objective* is more appropriate. Short-term objectives represent a logical breakdown of the major components of an annual goal, or may describe a precursor step or a building block skill. Objectives may be written to address targets in a successive (e.g., use single-symbol and then two-symbol messages), or an analogous (use three-symbol messages to comment during a structured activity) manner.

Session/Daily Targets

These refer to those behaviors or skills that are specifically targeted within a given day or activity. For example, during a game activity the student may be working on the key phrase, "My turn," whereas during a craft activity the student may be working on the phrase "Put here." Daily targets may be derivatives of the goals or short-term objective, or intermediary steps toward either. They encompass those skills the student is meant to accomplish within a given day, building toward the short-term objectives or long-term goals.

   The overarching goal of intervention is to facilitate acquisition of new skills. The sample goals presented in this chapter can be adapted accordingly to be written as annual goals, short-term/benchmark objectives, or even individual session targets. There are two daily data collection forms that can be downloaded from the accompanying website. The first one entitled, *Communicative Competency Goals Daily Data Collection Form* (Figure 6–2), provides a means for collecting data on target skills in each of the four competency areas. The other form entitled, *Daily Activities Data Collection Form* (Figure 6–3), lists target skills per activity. For example, during snack the student may be working on key phrases for requesting preferred food items (e.g., "I want more that.") and assistance with opening a container (e.g., "Can you open it?"), whereas during a shared reading activity, they may be working on key phrases to comment and/or respond to teacher-posed prompts (e.g., "I turn it," "It there," I like/don't like it"). At the bottom of this data collection form are spaces for documenting progress towards specific skills that are going to be targeted throughout the student's day (e.g., transitioning communication book between activities, greeting peers).

While the ultimate goal is to for the student to execute skills independently, it may be necessary to initially provide the student with support as a skill is emerging. In this instance, it is important to note the level of support required for the student to successfully execute the skill (e.g., "Student will use the two-symbol phrase 'My turn' given an adult-facilitated interaction between an activity involving one other student."). This allows you to document the student's gradual, but steady, progress toward independent mastery of specific skills. The following provides potential levels of support or prompts a student may benefit from as they move toward independence. Coding level of support is beneficial in documenting a student's progress. Examples of how these codes are applied are provided in the two data collection samples in Figures 6–2 and 6–3.

- **Mastered/Independent (+):** The student demonstrates target skill independently.
- **Natural/Environmental Cue (C):** The student demonstrates skill in response to a natural cue (e.g., student responds to peer's greeting, student requests desired object in response to a communication temptation).
- **Indirect Prompt (IP):** The student performs target skill in response to an indirect gestural or verbal prompt (e.g., "What do you need?" "Are you forgetting something?").
- **Direct Prompt (DP):** The student executes target skill in response to a direct verbal (e.g., "Get your communication book") or gestural prompt (e.g., communication guide points to communication book to encourage student to use it).
- **Model (M):** The student executes skill following a model. It can also be coded as a partial model (PM) if the student was able to demonstrate the skill following a partial model (e.g., communication guide models, "I want" and the student responds, "I want juice").

AAC Intervention: Communicative Competency Goals Daily Data Collection Form

Student's Name: _**Maggie**_   Date: _**7/14/2014**_   Communication Guide: _**Alicia**_

Linguistic Goal(s): Increase MNSM to 3.5; Use 15 new core vocabulary words, Expand sentence constructions

Daily Linguistic Targets:

Use 3 symbol messages	M	M	M	M	+	+	+	+	+	DP
	DP	IP	+	+	+	+	+	M	M	M
Use core vocabulary words: do, like, here	M	M	M	M	+	+	+	IP	IP	C
	IP	C	+	+	+	+	+	M		
Use sentence construction: actor-action-object	+	+	+	+	+	+	+	+	+	+
	IP	IP	+	+	+	+	+			

Operational Goal(s): Use 5 navigational tools, locate activity specific folders/pages, transition communication system

Daily Operational Targets:

Navigate to home/core vocabulary page	DP	DP	DP	IP	IP	IP	+	+	+	+
	+	+	IP	+	+					
Locate activity specific folder/page	+	+	+	+	DP	DP	DP	+	+	
Transition communication system	IP	IP	IP	IP	+	+	+	+	IP	

Strategic Goal(s): Recognize and respond to failed communication attempt; indicate completion of activity

Daily Strategic Targets:

Use communication tap to gain attention	H	H	H	H	M	M	+	+	+	IP
	+	+								
Use phrase all done upon completion of activity	M	IP	IP	+	+	IP				

Social Goal(s): Expand purposes for communicating

Daily Social Targets:

Behavioral regulation: Request action/objects	+	+	+	+	+	+	IP	C	C	C
	+	+								
Social interaction: Greet peers and familiar adults	M	M	M	+	+	+	IP	IP		
Joint Attention: Comment	M	M	+	+	+	+	M	IP	+	+
	+	+								

Rate of Initiations (I) and Responses (R)

Snack	I	I	I	I	R	R	I	I	I	R	R	I	I	R	I	I
Shared Story Activity	R	R	R	R	I	I	I	R	R	R	I	R				
Craft	R	R	I	I	I	R	R	I	R	I	I	R				

Comments: *Several new skills were introduced today which accounts for additional modeling and hand-over-hand prompting. Previously introduced and mastered skills were executed with greater level of independence. Maggie really enjoyed craft activity. More difficulty with transitions.*

PROMPT CODES: Independent (+), Natural/Environmental Cue (C), Indirect Prompt (IP), Direct Prompt (DP), Model (M), Hand-over-hand Model (H)

Figure 6–2. Communicative Competency Goals Daily Data Collection Form.

AAC Intervention: Daily Activities Data Collection Form

Student's Name: _____ *Connor* _____   Date: _7/12/2014_   Communication Guide: _*Amanda*_

Activity Specific Intervention Targets:

Activity: *Opening circle activity/story: "From Head to Toe" by Eric Carle*

I here (Part of daily routine)	+									
Can you _____? (Social: Joint Attention/Ask Question)	M	M	M	M	DP	DP	IP	IP		
I can do it! (Social: Joint Attention/Comment)	M	DP	IP	+	IP	+	+	+		
You do it! (Social: Behavioral Regulation/Request Action)	M	DP	IP	+	+	+	+	IP		

Activity: *Gross Motor-Scooter boards with occupational therapist*

My turn (Social: Social Interaction/Participate in Social Routine)	M	+	C	+	+	+	+			
You turn (Social: Behavioral Regulation/Request Action)	M	M	+	IP	+	+	+	+		
More go (Social: Behavioral Regulation/Request Action)	C	C	C	C	C	C	C			
Stop or no more go (Social: Behavioral Regulation/Request Action)	DP	DP	+	+	+	IP				

C: Communication guide stops pulling scooter board creating a communication temptation

Activity: *Snack*

I want juice/I want more juice (Social: Behavioral Regulation-Request Object)	+	+	+	+	+	+	+	+		
Open it (Social: Behavioral Regulation/Request Action)	M	M	M	IP	+	+	+			
I like it (Social: Joint Attention/Comment) New skill	M	M	M	M	M					
I don't like it (Social: Joint Attention/Comment)New Skill	M	M	M	M	M					

Activity: *Craft-Decorating picture frames*

I want + object (Social: Behavioral Regulation-Request Object)	C	C	C	C	+	+	+	+		
I want + color attribute + object (Social: Behavioral Regulation-Request Object)	M	C	C	C	C	C	+	+	+	+
Put here (Social: Joint Attention/Respond to Question)	+	+	+	+	+	+				
Not here (Social: Behavioral Regulation/Protest)	M	M	M	M	DP	IP	+			

C: Communication holds up a choice of objects or color options creating a communication temptation

Activity: *Bubble play with fan and nets*

Turn it on/off (Social: Behavioral Regulation/Request Action)	M	M	M	M	DP	DP	IP	+	+	+
I pop/ You pop (Social: Behavioral Regulation/Request Action)	M	M	IP	+	+	IP	+			
Make more bubbles (Social: Behavioral Regulation/Request Action)	M	M	M	M	M	M	IP	IP		
I got it (Social: Joint Attention/Comment)	M	M	M	M	M	IP	IP	IP	+	

Daily Intervention Targets:

Transition communication system (Operational)	IP	IP	IP	+	+	+	IP	+		
Greet peers (Social: Social Interaction/Greet)	IP	IP	IP	+	+	+	IP			
Use phrase "all done" upon completion of activity (Strategic)	M	M	M	+	+	+	IP	IP		
Locate activity specific folders (Operational)	+	+	+	IP	IP	+	+	+		
Use communication tap (Strategic)	H	H	H	H	M	M	DP	DP	IP	IP

Comments:

Connor had a great day. He was introduced to a lot of new linguistic/social targets. Independency on operational goals dependent on intrinsic motivation (e.g., snack)

PROMPT CODES: Independent (+), Natural/Environmental Cue (C), Indirect Prompt (IP), Direct Prompt (DP), Model (M), Hand-over-hand Model (H)

Figure 6–3. Daily Activities Data Collection Form.

◆ **Hand-over-hand Model (H):** The communication guide physically guides the student through the target skills placing their hand over the student's hand.

There are times when it is necessary to gather data on a student's overall response to the intervention and generalization of skills across activities and environments. Collecting a representative sample of the student's AAC use can provide a wealth of information across the different competency areas and can be used for reporting/establishing present levels of performance in general or documenting progress on specific skills. The following is a list of potential skills that may be recorded when sampling a student's AAC use.

Linguistic Targets:

◆ Total number of different symbols used by the student
◆ Total number of core vocabulary words
◆ Total number of fringe vocabulary words
◆ Mean number of symbols per message (MNSM)
◆ Inventory of language constructions

Social Targets:

◆ Inventory of communicative purposes
◆ Rate of initiations
◆ Rate of responses
◆ Ratio of initiations to responses

Operational Targets:

◆ Inventory of navigational tool skills (e.g., on/off, returning to home page, activating message bar)
◆ Description of AAC system (display type, number of cells)
◆ Independence of use (locating device when needed, transitioning device from activity to activity)

Strategic Targets:

◆ Response to communication breakdowns
◆ Multifunction word use

Gather a Representative Sample

It is important to gather a representative sample of the student's AAC use. In order to document an authentic account of the student's AAC use, it is essential to observe the student across multiple environments, activities, and days. It is not uncommon for different activities to elicit different types of communicative acts, language constructions, and vocabulary. As communicators, our communicative acts (e.g., requesting, commenting, protesting) reflect our conversational role (e.g., initiator versus responder) relative to the given activity. In one activity, an individual may assume the primary role of responder, such as during a shared reading experience, responding to teacher prompted questions, whereas a different activity, in this instance snack, may give an individual a greater opportunity to initiate communication attempts. In order to have a representative sample of the student's AAC use, it may be necessary to enlist the assistance of the classroom teacher or paraprofessionals who have been properly trained.

Record

Record the student's responses verbatim using the *Communication Sampling Form* (Figure 6–4). Each response is recorded and the communicative purpose is coded. It is useful to know what specific symbols a student is using; therefore, it is important to not only record the student's messages but the specific symbols used to construct those messages. For example, if "I want" or "My turn" are represented as single symbols then they are coded as such (e.g., I–want) using a dash mark to indicate they are represented as a single symbol. On the other hand, if "I want" is represented by the separate symbols, "I" and "want" (likewise "My turn" is represented by the individual symbols "My" and "turn"), it is coded as two symbols (e.g., I/want) separated by a back slash mark. Refer to Figure 6–4 for an illustration of this concept.

Code Communicative Intent

Beginning communicators use communication for three broad purposes: behavior regulation, social interaction, and joint attention, with subcategories within each of these categories. Each communicative message is coded for its communicative intent (e.g., Behavioral Regulation-Request Action). It is possible that a single message may serve dual functions, depending on the context. Therefore it is necessary to consider the context in which the message was used before determining the student's communicative intent of the message. Prior to observing the student, review *Definitions of Communicative Functions* (Appendix 6–A), or download a copy from the accompanying website and keep it readily available for easy reference.

Record Discourse Role

Record the discourse role of each communicative message as either an initiation (I) or response (R) and what level of support the student required (see previous section) to successfully execute the skill. If a student uses the identical phrase repeatedly in a sequence, only record it once, unless the child uses the same phrase for a different communicative function. For example,

Communication Unit	Transcription	Number of symbols
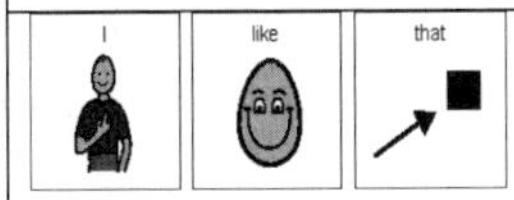	I/like/that	3
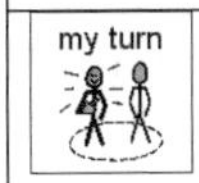	My-turn	1
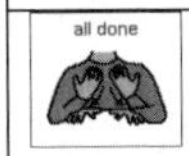	All-done	1
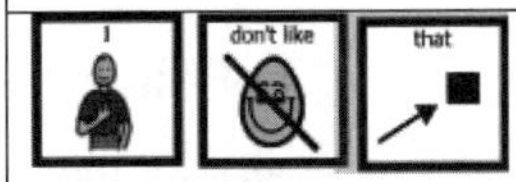	I/don't like/that	3
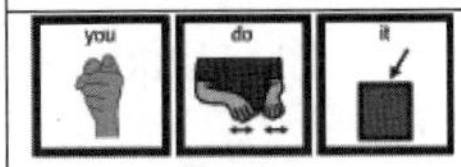	You/do/it	3
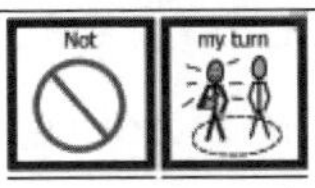	Not/my-turn	2
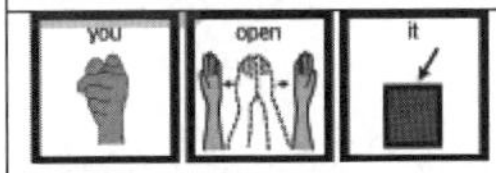	You/open/it	3
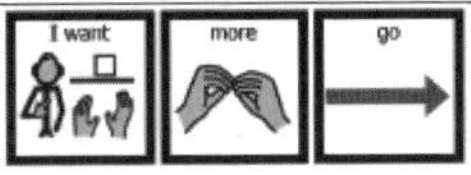	I-want/more/go	3

Figure 6–4. Transcribing Communication Units.

a student may use the phrase "I don't like" as a response to a question, to indicate a preference, or to protest. See Table 6–5.

Analyze Data

Once a representative sample has been collected, recorded, and coded, the next step involves analyzing the data across the four competency areas. The *AAC Competency Skills Progress Report* (Figure 6–5), which can be downloaded in its entirety from the accompanying website, provides a summative means for reporting critical data and structure in how to examine the student's AAC use across the four competency areas. Each section of the summary report will be discussed in detail.

Table 6–5. Examples of Identifying Discourse Role, Number of Symbols per Message, Language Construction and Communicative Functions

	Discourse Role	Number of Symbols per Message	Language Construction	Communicative Function
I/here	R	2	Actor-Location	JA-Comment
Can/you/turn/it?	I	4	Action-Actor-Actor-Object	JA-Ask Question
I/can/do/it	I	4	Actor-Action-Action-Object	JA-Comment
You/do/it	I	3	Actor-Action-Object	BR-Request Action
My/turn	I	2	Possession-Object	SI-Participate in Social Routine
Your/turn	I	2	Actor-Action	BR-Request Action
More/go	I	2	Determine-Action	BR-Request Action
I/want/more/go	I	4	Actor-Action-Determiner-Action	BR-Request Action
No/go	I	2	Negation-Action	BR-Protest
I/want/juice	I	3	Actor-Action-Object	BR-Request Object
I/want/cracker	I	3	Actor-Action-Object	BR-Request Object
I/want/popcorn	I	3	Actor-Action-Object	BR-Request Object
Open/juice	I	2	Action-Object	BR-Request Action
I/want/red/cracker	I	4	Actor-Action-Attribute-Object	BR-Request Object
Put/here	R	2	Action-Location	JA-Respond to Question
Not/here	R	2	Negation-Location	JA-Respond to Question
Turn/on	R	2	Action-Preposition	BR-Request Action
I/pop/bubble	I	3	Actor-Action-Object	JA-Comment
Make/more	I	2	Action-Determine	BR-Request Action
I/got/it	I	3	Actor-Action-Object	JA-Comment
Hi	I	1	Misc.	SI-Greet
All done	I	1	Misc.	JA-Comment

Discourse Role: R-Responder; I-Initiator.

Name: __Connor__   Date of Report: __July 2014/End of Summer Session__

LINGUISTIC SKILLS

Symbol Inventory:

I	here	can	do	it	book	my	turn	more	go
like	don't/not	want	cracker	juice	popcorn	cookie	cup	paper	red
green	blue	jewel	sticker	put	on	off	make	pop	bubbles
got	all done	yellow							

Symbol Knowledge:

TOTAL NUMBER DIFFERENT WORDS: ___33___   CORE VOCABULARY: ___17___   FRINGE VOCABULARY: ___16___

Mean Number of Symbols per Message (MNSM):

Total Number of Symbols	Total Number of Communicative Messages	MNSM
58	23	2.5

Message Constructions:

I want + preferred food items/objects	M	Mastered (+)
I want + color attribute + preferred food items/objects	E	Student uses the sentence construction independently and frequently
Action + Object	E	Emerging (E)
Negation + Action	E	Student uses the sentence construction with *moderate support* such as indirect prompt or initial model
Actor + Location	E	Learning (L)
Action + Location	E	Student uses sentence construction with *significant support* such as direct prompting, modeling and hand-over-hand prompting
Action + Object	E	
Actor + Action + Object	E	

OPERATIONAL SKILLS

Briefly describe student's AAC system: Connor is using a Mini iPad with the Proloquo2go app. His home page consists of 36 cells, giving him access to 30 core words (17 are currently used on a regular basis) and six activity folders. He independently access two of these folders (snack, preferred items).

Navigational Skills:

	Independently	With Some Support	With Significant Support
Turn on/off device	X		
Activate message bar		X	
Return to home/core page		X	
Transition communication system through day		X	
Find activity specific folders/pages/vocabulary strips		X	

Figure 6–5. AAC Competency Skills Progress Report. *continues*

SOCIAL SKILLS

Communicative Functions:

BEHAVIOR REGULATION	60%	SOCIAL INTERACTION	15%	JOINT ATTENTION	25%
Request Objects (RO)	Frequently	Request Social Routine	Occasionally	Comment	Occasionally
Request Action (RA)	Frequently	Greet	Occasionally	Ask Question	Occasionally
Protest (P)	Occasionally	Show Off	Never	Respond to Question	Occasionally
		Call	Never	Share Experience	Never
		Request Permission	Never	Label	Never
		Acknowledgement	Never		
		Complete Verbal Script	Occasionally		

Responses and Initiations:

Activity: Snack			Activity: Shared Reading			Activity: Craft		
Total # Responses	Total # Initiations	Total # Responses	Total # Responses	Total # Initiations	Total # Responses	Total # Responses	Total # Initiations	Total # Responses
18	14	4	8	2	6	11	5	6

STRATEGIC SKILLS

Communication Repairs:

Given a failed communication attempt the student...	Independently	With Some Support	With Significant Support
Repeats messages			X
Gains communication partner's attention and repeats message			X
Revises message			X

Replacement Behaviors:

Student replaces aberrant forms of communication (e.g., eloping, shutting down) with more acceptable forms of communication:	Independently	With Some Support	With Significant Support
Requests help		X	
Indicate needs for break		X	
Indicates completion of an activity or task (e.g., "all done")		X	

Multifunction Word Use:

Core Word	Example of Use 1	Example of Use 2	Example of Use 3
Turn	My turn (object)	I turn it (action)	

Comments:

Figure 6–5. *continued*

Linguistic Targets

It is important to monitor a student's symbolic knowledge, their use and understanding of symbols, both from a quantitative angle, as well as a qualitative perspective. By identifying a student's symbolic inventory you can ascertain the total number of different symbols they are using and compare how many of those symbols represent core vocabulary and how many represent fringe words.

Symbol Inventory. After gathering a representative sample of the student's AAC use, create an inventory of the different symbols the student used throughout the sample. To avoid inflating the student's true inventory, do not include words/symbols the student uses on a single basis or for a specific activity, but rather include words they use on a regular, even semiregular basis. Identifying the symbols a student uses is important for two reasons. First, it is a relatively easy way to evaluate and monitor a student's progression related to their symbolic knowledge. Secondly, it gives you an indication of which symbols on their device they are using and which ones they are not using. This translates into two actions on your part: (1) teach them how to use the symbols they are not accessing, or (2) remove those symbols from their device and add ones they are more likely to use.

Total Number of Different Symbols (TNDS). Calculating the student's TNDS provides a quantitative means to describe the student's symbol knowledge and can be easily compared to previous or future inventories.

Core Vocabulary Set Versus Fringe Vocabulary Words. Of particular interest to the intervention described in this book is to develop a student's understanding and use of core vocabulary; therefore, is it important to continually monitor how a student is expanding his or her knowledge in this area. Utilizing the symbol inventory, note (suggest using different color highlight markers) symbols that represent core vocabulary from those that represent fringe vocabulary terms.

Mean Number of Symbols per Message (MNSM). Similar to a mean length of utterance (MLU) calculation, MNSM is an objective quantitative means to evaluate the student's linguistic progression, in this instance as it relates to AAC use. The MSNM is calculated by adding up the total number of symbols used within the sample and then dividing it by the total number of messages. Messages that are elicited in response to a model or those messages in which the student is prompted (e.g., through pointing) to use specific symbols are not calculated in determining the MNSM. As well, messages that are repeatedly used by the student are only credited a single occurrence in the MNSM calculation. Calculating the MNSM may not be appropriate or possible to measure with all AAC apps/device, or may need to be interpreted within the context of a specific program/app itself.

Message Constructions. It is possible that students will not demonstrate a significant increase in MNSM within a specific time frame, but that should not be misinterpreted as a lack of linguistic advancement. Although not exhibiting a vertical improvement, moving from using MNSM of 2.5 to 3.7, some students may exhibit improvements on a horizontal trajectory. In this instance, they expand the types of sentence constructions they are using in composing their messages. Using the communication sample, compile a list of sentence construction (e.g., actor-action-object) describing level of proficiency as *mastered, emerging, or learning*. Although the message "I want juice" (or reference to other object or preferred activity) is an example of an actor-action-object sentence, it is reported as its own construction. This specific message construction is often one of the first messages children master well before they use actor-action-object constructions with a wide range of actors, actions, and objects. Refer to Linguistic Skills Portion of the *AAC Competency Skills Progress Report* (see Figure 6–5) for examples of how linguistic skills can be reported.

Operational Targets

In this section you will not only be describing specific skills demonstrated by the student, but also providing a description of their current AAC system (e.g., number of cells, size of cells, number of core vocabulary). As a student's AAC system is customized to keep pace with their AAC skills, it is therefore a strong indicator of their progress. The following are examples of some of the skills and AAC features you may want to describe in documenting a student's progress.

Description of AAC System. As previously stated, a student's AAC system is changed as the student's needs change and skills develop. Therefore, describing a student's AAC system and how it has been changed or modified to meet the student's expanding communication needs is another way to document student's overall progress. The following are some of the aspects of changes to an AAC system that will demonstrate the student user's growth. *Type of display*: Describe the type of display they are using. Are they using a static, dynamic, or hybrid display system? Are there certain activities or environments in which they are using a scene display? Students frequently begin with a static, even non-technology-based communication system, but as their skills and communication needs change, so does the ACC system. *Number of cells per page:* Record the number of cells per page. *Number of pages/folders:* How many and what types of folders is the student using on a regular basis (e.g., snack folder, preferred activities, classroom materials, outside playground activities)?

Inventory of Navigational Skills. This area of proficiency examines the student's skills related to the operational use of their AAC system. The inventory includes skills related to turning on/off their system, adjusting volume, deleting previous messages, navigating back to the home page, activating the message bar, and locating pages based on need. The *AAC Competency Skills Progress Report* (see Figure 6–5) provides a list of skills that can be recorded as exhibited *independently, with some support, with significant support*. If the student can execute a particular skill with independence on 90% of the opportunities, they are considered *independent* on that particular skill. If they can demonstrate the skill with natural cues (C) or indirect prompts (IP), then they are considered proficient in that particular skill *with some support*. If the student continues to benefit from direct prompting (DP), modeling (M), and even hand-over-hand modeling (H), their proficiency is established *with significant support*.

Transitioning AAC System. It is important for the student to take ownership of their communication system and be responsible for having it with them throughout their day. Refer to the Operational Skills Portion of the *AAC Competency Skills Progress Report* (see Figure 6–5) for examples of how operational skills can be reported.

Social Targets

This is a very important aspect of the intervention approach described in this book: expanding students' purposes for communicating and increasing the frequency of communication acts. This intervention approach strives to teach students to communicate beyond purposes of requesting preferred food items and activities, therefore it is critical to monitor their progress in this area of competency.

Identify Communicative Purposes. Based on the communication sample, calculate an estimate of the student's use of their communication across the three broad purposes of communication (i.e., behavior regulation, social interaction, joint attention). For each subcategory within each broad category, estimate frequency, reporting them as occurring *frequently, occasionally, never*. The following is an example of how this area of functioning may be reported.

> *Based on a sample gathered over the course of three regular school days, Charlie used communication for three broad purposes: behavior regulation, social interaction, and joint attention. Sixty percent of his communication attempts were for the purposes of regulating the behavior of others, 15% for the purposes of social interaction, and 25% for purposes related to joint attention. Of his behavior regulatory acts, he used communication to frequently request objects and actions, and occasionally to protest. For purposes of social interaction, Charlie used communication to request social*

> *routines, greet peers, and complete verbal scripts. He has yet to demonstrate social interaction types of communicative exchanges to show off, call attention, request permission, or acknowledge. Charlie establishes joint attention primarily through commenting and asking and answering questions. He does not currently share experiences or labels items in his environment for the purposes of establishing joint attention.*

Compute Rate of Initiations and Responses. As previously mentioned in Chapter 3, AAC users are less likely to initiate communication, usually assuming the discourse role of responders (Beukelman & Mirenda, 2013) in the conversation. In addition to increasing rate of initiations, it is important to increase overall rate of communicating. This can be evaluated by examining the rate of initiations and responses over 5-minute blocks. During predetermined activities such as opening circle, snack, tabletop activity (e.g., craft), document the number of communicative acts observed within 5-minute blocks, coding each act as either a responses or initiation. To ensure an authentic account of a student's progress from one reporting period to the next, it is important to note the number of communicative acts during similar activities. Refer to the Social Skills Portion of the *AAC Competency Skills Progress Report* (see Figure 6–5), for examples of how social skills can be reported.

Strategic Competence

Communication Repairs. One of the shortcomings of any AAC system is a communication attempt being ignored or misinterpreted. This is compounded in students with CCNs who may not even recognize when a communication attempt was missed, or those students who lack the persistence in conveying their very important message by either simply repeating the message alone, gaining their communication partner's attention by using an acceptable means such as tapping them on the shoulder and then restating their original message, or revising what they've said so it is more easily understood. Some students with CCNs, perhaps because of ongoing experience with failed communication, actually become somewhat passive and have to be taught how to be persistent in their communication attempts.

Replacement of Aberrant Communicative Behaviors. Too often, children with CCNs use aberrant, socially undesirable behaviors such as biting, screaming, hitting, tantruming, or avoidance, such as eloping to indicate when a task is too hard, being unmotivated, or expressing a general displeasure with the current situation. One goal of introducing AAC to a child who uses undesirable behaviors as a means of communication, is to replace these socially undesirable behaviors with ones that are more socially acceptable.

Requests that can be challenging for the student to communicate (without exhibiting undesirable behavior) include the need to request assistance or a break. Similar to the communication repairs, more appropriate forms of communication are noted as executed with *independence, some support, or significant support.*

Multifunction Word Use. One of the biggest limitations of any AAC system is a lack of access to an infinite vocabulary set. For early communicators, access to vocabulary is even more limited. In this area of functioning, it is important to notice how the student is compensating for such limitations. The most obvious one is to examine their multifunction word use, that is, their ability to use a single term for multiple purposes. Refer to the Strategic Skills Portion of the *AAC Competency Skills Progress Report* (see Figure 6–5) for examples of how strategic skills can be reported.

PROGRESS MONITORING: AN ESSENTIAL COMPONENT OF THE INTERVENTION PROCESS

This book describes AAC intervention as a process, with progress monitoring as an essential component. Progress monitoring begins during the **assessment phase** by gathering information from a variety of resources to establish PLOPs across the four competency areas. From this information, during the **intervention-planning phase**, goals are established in the areas of linguistic, operational, social, and strategic competence. Throughout the **intervention implementation phase**, the student's response is strategically monitored so that revisions, alterations, and modifications can be made to either their communication system or the intervention itself to ensure steady progress continues. The process of monitoring progress is one important piece of the intervention process that will allow teams to keep a student moving forward in the quest for communicative competence.

REFERENCES

Beukelman, D. R., & Mirenda, P. (2013). *Augmentative and alternative communication: Supporting children and adults with complex communication needs* (4th ed.). Baltimore, MD: Paul Brookes.
Dodd, J. L., & Gorey, M. (2014). AAC intervention as an immersion model. *Communication Disorders Quarterly, 35*(2), 103–107. http://dx.doi.org/10.1177/1525740113504242
Doran, G. T. (1981). There's a S.M.A.R.T. way to write management's goals and objectives. *Management Review, 70*(11), 35–36.
Individuals with Disabilities Education Act, 20 U.S.C. § 1400. (2004).

APPENDIX 6–A
Definitions of Categories of Communicative Functions

Category	Definitions	Discourse Structure	Examples
		BEHAVIORAL REGULATION	
Request Object (RO)	Acts or utterances used to demand a desired tangible object. Includes requesting consumable and non-consumable items.	AAC user requests object and waits to receive desired object.	I want XXX, want more, want that, yes (in response to question prompt—"Do you want?"), I need glue, more bubbles
Request action (RA)	Acts or utterances used to command another person to carry out an action. Includes requesting assistance and other actions involving another person or between another person and an object.	AAC user requests action and waits for response	Open, you push, you go, I go, read it, I need help, you do it, make go, more go, come here, again, do it again, turn, you turn
Protest (PR)	Acts or utterances used to command another to cease an undesired action. Includes resisting another's action and rejection of object that is offered.	AAC user protests and waits for response.	No, stop it, no go, no turn, no want, I don't like, no read
		SOCIAL INTERACTION	
Greet	Acts or utterances used to gain another's attention to indicate notice of their presence. Includes greetings, calling, and conversational devices such as politeness markers and boundary markers.	AAC user makes a comment and may or may not wait for response. Non AAC user makes a comment (or act) and AAC user follows up with an appropriate response	Child waves or says "Hi" when adult enters the room. Child shouts "Mom" when his mother is across the room to get her attention. Child gives the adult a kiss or says "Thank you" after the adult gave a desired object to the child, "Bye," I here"

Category	Definitions	Discourse Structure	Examples
Participation in a social routine (RS)	Acts or utterances used to command another to commence or continue carrying out a game or social interaction. Acts or utterances used to participate in a game or social routine. This specific type of action request involves an interaction between another person and the AAC user usually centered around a game or fun oriented/social interaction.	AAC user makes a request or comment and waits for response	Want chase, you do it, my turn, your turn, you go, I go
Showing-off (S)	Acts used to attract attention to something or something they are doing in an effort to say, "look at me"	AAC user addresses person (not object) and waits for response.	Look here, I did it!
Request permission (RP)	Acts or utterances used to seek another's consent to carry out an action.	AAC user requests consent, waits for a response, and then responds by carrying out the action.	I turn, I go potty, I do it, glue on?
Completion of a Verbal Script	Acts or utterances used to complete a verbal script	Non-AAC user provides a verbal script leaving off the final word or phrase and AAC user completes the script	Ready, set, GO or 1, 2, THREE, Take it OFF

continues

Appendix 6–A. *continued*

Category	Definitions	Discourse Structure	Examples
JOINT ATTENTION			
Comment (C)	Acts or utterances used to direct another's attention to an object or event. Includes showing, describing, informing, and interactive labeling.	AAC user makes a comment directed toward an object or event, may or may not wait for a response.	I like that, I don't like that, I feel bad/good, no like (commenting not protesting, sharing a preference), no (in response to "do you like?")
Ask Question	Utterances used to find out something about an object or event. Includes wh-questions and other utterances having the intonation contour of an interrogative.	AAC user asks a question and waits for response.	What that? Where go? Do you like play?
Respond to Question	Acts or utterances in response to a question posed by another.	Non-AAC user asks a question and AAC user responds	Responds to "What is that?" "What's your name?" Does not include responding to question request (e.g., "Do you want cookie?") or prompt question to retell past event or share upcoming event.
Share a past or future experience	Acts or utterances to retell a past experience or notify about an upcoming experience	AAC user makes comment and may nor may not wait for response.	I go movie, I eat that I go lunch

Source: Adapted from Wetherby, A., & Prutting, C. (1984). Profiles of communicative and cognitive-social abilities in autistic children. *Journal of Speech and Hearing Research, 27,* 364–377; and Wetherby, A. M., Cain, D. H., Yonclas, D. G., & Walker, V. G. (1988). Analysis of intentional communication of normal children from the prelinguistic to the multiword stage. *Journal of Speech and Hearing Research, 31,* 240–252.

CHAPTER 7

Case Examples

The eight student case examples presented in this chapter illustrate the implementation of the intervention program described in this book. Key aspects of the intervention process will be highlighted throughout each case example. The students in these case examples represent children with a range of diagnoses and disorders, each with their own unique set of communication needs. As stated earlier, the intervention approach described in this book was not developed with any single AAC system in mind, but rather developed as an approach and process that has universal appeal across systems and devices. The case examples will demonstrate how the intervention approach can be applied with students who are using high-tech communication systems, as well as with those who use low-tech communication systems, such as communication boards and books.

The students presented in these case examples all participated in the intervention disguised under the ruse of "camp" as a component of their extended school year (ESY) programs. ESY refers to services that are provided to students with exceptional needs during an extended break (e.g., summer) to prevent the irrevocable loss of skills that is likely to occur during a lengthy period of time without services (Individuals with Disabilities Act [IDEA], 2004). The case examples will also provide additional models of how to write present levels of performance (PLOPs) and goals. Embedded within each case example are suggestions on how to prompt/teach new skills, along with strategies for facilitating continued progression.

HOW TO USE THIS CHAPTER

The purpose of this chapter is to provide specific examples of how this approach is adapted to meet the needs of students with varying needs and AAC systems. Each case example will provide sample language for reporting PLOPs, along with goals to address the needs in each of the four competency areas: linguistic competence, operational competence, social competence, and strategic competence. Each case example provides an overall summary of the student's response to the intervention, including strategies/recommendations to facilitate further acquisition of AAC use.

Assessment Phase: Establishing PLOPs and Baselines

Prior to the implementation of the two-week intensive intervention program, present levels of performance (PLOPs) were established in each of the four competency areas. Baseline performance of related skills were identified through review of each student's confidential file, observations of the student in a variety of environments, administration of standardized tests, and completion of formalized observational checklists of both the targeted student and students of a similar age or developmental level. The purpose of establishing baseline skills and reporting PLOPs was threefold. First, the information gathered during this pre-intervention process was utilized to develop a comprehensive picture of the student's current means of communication, including its benefits and limitations in meeting the student's communication needs. Secondly, areas of need were identified in each of the four competency areas, and intervention targets (e.g., goals) were developed accordingly. Lastly, it was important to recognize the student's strengths and weaknesses so that intervention techniques and participation expectations could be customized to optimize each student's response to the intervention.

The assessment phase of the intervention process (Chapter 3) focused on gathering critical information to be applied during the intervention-planning phase (Chapter 4) in order to customize each student's communication system and develop lessons to facilitate their use of communication for an expanding range of purposes. The data collection began with a review of the students' assessment reports and their previous individualized educational programs (IEPs). As is common, many of the students who were considered ideal candidates for this intervention approach (refer to Chapter 2 regarding "Who could benefit from this type of intervention") had been exposed to a myriad of interventions with mixed results, and the students in these eight case studies were no exception. Knowing how students responded to different approaches (e.g., PECS, functional communication training) was critical in blending the successes of those approaches, while recognizing their limitations in building upon the student's communication skills.

Through observation, review of relevant documents, administrations of criterion-referenced/standardized tests (e.g., Test of Aided Symbol Performance), and informal probes, skills related to AAC use were identified. In addition to gathering information regarding physical abilities related to AAC use, necessary information was gathered regarding each student's capabilities in the areas of cognition, language, literacy, and sensory perception. Although the purpose of assessment was not to necessarily make recommendations regarding a particular AAC system, the information collected was critical to customizing the student's current AAC system and developing a communication system to optimize their learning potential. Additionally, students were observed in various activities, both structured and unstructured, in their regular classroom(s) throughout their day to observe participation patterns and identify communication needs.

Upon conclusion of gathering the data, clear descriptions of each student's current communication abilities, needs, and abilities related to AAC usage (e.g., access abilities, understanding of icons) were established so that a communication system could be adapted or created to support the student's progression toward communicative competence.

Intervention Planning Phase

During the intervention-planning phase of these eight case studies, time was dedicated to developing or customizing each student's communication system, and engineering the environment to optimize learning opportunities. For those students already using AAC systems, the manner in which their devices were programmed (e.g., limited access to core vocabulary, preprogrammed messages) often was an obstacle to facilitating their use of communication for an expanding range of purposes (e.g., commenting, asking questions) and/or their ability to create novel sentence patterns. Therefore, those students' AAC systems were reconfigured to give greater access to core vocabulary, which enabled the ability to create novel sentence patterns and extend communicative acts beyond requesting preferred food items and objects. An AAC system was developed for those students who did not currently have one. Visual supports, such as visual schedules, adapted stories, and choice boards were incorporated throughout the environment to create an immersive environment, which provided the students with multiple opportunities to experience their language system in meaningful contexts.

Additionally, during the intervention planning phase, communication guides were trained in the principles of the intervention approach, and their roles in the intervention process was defined. Communication guides developed an understanding of the facets of communication (e.g., communicative competence, communicative functions). They learned the impact of teaching core vocabulary to facilitate communicative competence. They received instruction and practice in applying various language-enhancing strategies (i.e., modeling, self-talk, expansionism, and parallel talk) utilizing aided modeling techniques (e.g., aided language stimulation) to foster the acquisition of communication. Finally, they learned how to scaffold and create communication opportunities throughout the students' day.

Another piece of the intervention-planning phase was the establishment of intervention targets. For each student, a minimum of one goal was identified in each competency area (i.e., linguistic, operational, social, and strategic). Identifying desired outcomes was necessary to provide an objective means for evaluating each student's response to the intervention.

Intervention Implementation Phase

Each of the students presented in this chapter received a total of 24 to 30 hours of intense intervention distributed over the course of two weeks within the context of both structured and non-structured activities. Each intervention session began with one-on-one time between the student and his/her communication guide which transitioned into a structured opening activity (e.g., opening circle). Each session concluded with one-on-one time with their communication guide to update their "school-to-home" communication book (refer to Chapter 4 regarding the importance of a "school-to-home" communication book and how to create one) and closing activity (e.g., "Good Bye Song"). Throughout the three-hour intervention session students were engaged in a variety of large and small group activities including story time, craft, snack, and gross motor activities. Students were given an opportunity to learn/participate in typical playground type games/activities. The following is a summary of the students presented in this chapter:

- ◆ Case Example #1: 4-year, 11-month-old male with primary eligibility of autism and a secondary eligibility of speech-language impairment using a communication book.
- ◆ Case Example #2: 7-year-old male with primary eligibility of autism using an iPad with the Proloquo2go app.
- ◆ Case Example #3: 3-year, 9-month-old male with a primary diagnosis of speech-language impairment secondary to prenatal drug exposure using a no-tech flip-book communication system.
- ◆ Case Example #4: 15-year-old female with primary eligibility of autism and a secondary eligibility of intellectual disability using an iPad with the Speak For Yourself app.
- ◆ Case Example #5: 9-year, 2-month-old male with diagnoses of severe apraxia of speech, autism and intellectual disability using a communication board.
- ◆ Case Example #6: 5-year, 1-month-old male with delays in expressive language secondary to a diagnosis of cerebral palsy using the Accent 800 with the Unity Language System.
- ◆ Case Example # 7: 5-year, 4-month-old female with a primary eligibility of autism and a secondary eligibility of speech-language impairment using a communication book.
- ◆ Case Example #8 is 12-year, 10-month-old male with a primary diagnosis of autism using an iPad with the Speak for Yourself app.

CASE EXAMPLE #1: CONNOR

Connor, a 4-year, 11-month-old male, presents with a primary eligibility of autism and a secondary eligibility of specific language impairment (SLI). His primary language is English and it is the only language spoken in the home.

At the time of the intervention, Connor was enrolled in a preschool special day class specifically designed to meet the unique learning style of children with autism. In addition to his classroom placement, Connor received related services in the areas of speech-language intervention and occupational therapy. Speech and language IEP goals focused on requesting items necessary to complete a task, using a short phrase to describe a photo, and marking final consonants in single words and producing both consonants in blends (e.g. /sp/).

Means of Communication

Connor used verbal language, gestures, and a picture exchange communication book for the purposes of requesting preferred items. Verbal language consisted of the carrier phrase 'I want" + preferred food items, objects, and activities. A considerable area of challenge for Connor was initiating communication independently without prompting or direct modeling. Connor inconsistently labeled a few common objects within in his immediate environment Receptively, Connor comprehended simple, familiar routine-based one-step commands (e.g., "Get your backpack/lunch," "Show me ____") and identified common household and classroom objects, action words, shapes and animals. He participated in classroom routines and structured activities.

AAC Use and Experience

Prior to participating in the intervention program, Connor had experience using a picture exchange communication book consisting of the following picture icons: I want, I want break, all done, and a total of 10 picture icons for preferred food items and primary reinforcers. Given a gestural prompt to use his communication notebook, Connor would create the sentence strip "I want" + preferred food item/primary reinforcer to request during snack and lunch or upon completion of non-preferred activities/tasks. If his communication partner failed to respond to his requests he would sit quietly in his chair until he was prompted to try again.

Intervention

When introducing Connor to new phrases his communication guide used hand-over-hand modeling to guide Connor through his communication system. After two or three models Connor independently formulated the newly introduced two- to three-symbol messages. Connor was observed 100% of the time pairing verbal language with touching symbols. To support his participation during the opening and closing circle activities Connor was provided with a laminated strip of symbols with key phrases specific to the circle routines (e.g., "Hello" "Good Morning" "Bye"). After three models,

Connor was greeting his peers independently. Throughout the intervention Connor was provided with corrective feedback to encourage expansion of his utterances and acquisition of novel phrases.

Description of Communication System

Connor's communication system consisted of a communication board giving him access to 47 core vocabulary words represented in pictorial form and interchangeable activity-based fringe pages each composed of approximately 10 fringe word picture symbols, which varied depending on the activity, on a separate page. Refer to Table 7–1 for a summary of Connor's response to the intervention.

Response to Intervention

Connor demonstrates willingness to learn and express multiple novel phrases daily following initial models and prompts to use his communication book. Connor actively participated and attended to various classroom activities lasting up to 30 minutes in length using his communication board as a visual cue to facilitate the use of oral language. Following an initial model and practice provided by his communication guide Connor used his communication book accurately pointing to picture symbols while simultaneously verbalizing phrases. He expanded the purposes for which he communicates to include requesting actions, protesting, greeting and commenting. Connor was provided with an opportunity to explore the iPad programmed with the Proloquo2Go application. Connor demonstrated the ability to navigate the application and sequence pictures to formulate utterances for the purposes of requesting, however, he exhibited less simultaneous verbalization when using the iPad.

Suggestions and Recommendations

Connor was responsive to the implementation of a communication board as he was an active participant in every activity, both structured and unstructured. Connor accepted corrective feedback from his communication guide, which led to success in expanding his mean message length and expressing novel phrases. An additional component of the intervention per the request of his family and his current SLP was to explore the use of the iPad as a communication option for Connor. Connor demonstrated the ability to use an iPad and could benefit from its use. It is recommended that the IEP team consider this as an option for him in the future with the ultimate goal, regardless of the communication system (iPad or communication book), to focus on teaching Connor to communicate for an expanding range of communicative purposes.

Table 7–1. Summary of Connor's Response to the Intervention

PLOPs	Intervention Targets	Progress
Connor verbalizes the carrier phrases "*I want* ___" and "*I see* ___." Using a picture exchange communication system and following a gestural prompt to use his communication book, Connor constructs the sentence "I want" + preferred food items and primary reinforcers to regulate the behavior of another person.	Connor will express 3 novel phrases (e.g., I make ___," "I go ___") when given a communication temptation by verbalizing or touching symbols on his communication board no less than 10 times per day (*Linguistic*).	Connor points to picture symbols on his communication board simultaneously verbalizing to express various 2 to 4 word sentences for commenting (e.g., ("I like it"), requesting (e.g., " want| more|___"), greeting (e.g., "Hello good morning"), and protesting (e.g., "No thank you I want|___") following an initial model at the beginning of the current activity. Connor learned 2 to 3 novel phrases per activity and expressed them approximately 10 times per activity.
Connor is currently prompted (i.e., verbal prompt, "Get your book," paired with a gesture) to get his communication book when it is time for snack.	Connor will independently transition his communication board with him to various classroom activities (*Operational*).	Connor independently transitioned his communication board with him approximately three times per day to various classroom activities. Given a non-descript prompt (i.e., standing there waiting for him, 50% of the time paired with a visual gaze at his book) he transitioned his book the remainder of the opportunities.
Connor exhibits difficulty initiating social interactions without a communication temptation present. Connor initiates communication attempts given maximal verbal and physical cuing.	Connor will formulate and initiate 2- to 3-word phrases to make requests by touching 2 to 3 symbols on his communication board 10 times per day during classroom activities (*Social*).	Connor independently initiated requests for objects needed to complete classroom activities (e.g., craft activities) through verbalization using his communication board as a visual cue no less than 15 times per day. He independently initiated requests for actions when interacting with staff and peers by pointing to symbols on his communication board simultaneously verbalizing the phrase, "I want my turn please" approximately 15 times per day.

continues

Table 7–1. *continued*

PLOPs	Intervention Targets	Progress
When Connor's communication attempts are not responded to, he will engage in giggling behavior or get out of his seat. He has difficulty initiating his needs for assistance or gaining attention of staff without prompts.	Given a failed communication attempt, Connor will appropriately gain the attention of the appropriate person (peer or familiar adult) and restate his message on 4 out of 5 opportunities (*Strategic*).	Connor demonstrated difficulty recognizing a failed communication attempt. Given physical prompting (i.e., slightly raising elbow) and repetitive practice, Connor tapped the appropriate person on the arm to gain their attention.

The following suggestions are strategies to increase Connor's acquisition of receptive language and communication:

♦ Model novel phrases using picture symbols on an AAC system (e.g., communication board) as a visual aid.
♦ Model longer phrases using his AAC system (e.g., communication board) pairing verbal models with symbols on his communication system.
♦ Encourage Connor to use his communication board when he is exhibiting difficulty initiating interactions.
♦ Provide opportunities for expressive and receptive language development by asking him questions while reading stories to him using his communication book for visual support.
♦ Model ways for him to participate in shared reading experiences through the use of his communication book.
♦ Increase opportunities for social engagement by providing him with picture symbols (e.g., symbols of key words phrases affixed by a clip for ready access) to facilitate his use of polite conventions (e.g., "Hello," and "Goodbye") and comments to interact with others (e.g., "Good job").
♦ Provide corrective feedback encouraging him to repeat the utterance.

CASE EXAMPLE #2: EMILIO

Emilio, a seven-year-old boy, presents with a eligibility of autism spectrum disorder and qualifies for special education services under the eligibility of "autistic-like characteristics." In addition to being enrolled in a first grade special education class specifically designed for students with autism, he receives speech-language intervention services and the support of an in-class instructional aide. Goals are written in his IEP to support his development of communication through the use of an AAC system and to expand his understanding of language. Specifically, goals are written to increase his understanding and use of object labels and action words, increase his use of communication for the purposes of requesting preferred objects and continuation of preferred activities to replace aberrant means of communication (e.g., behavior). Goals related to speech sound production focus on improving production through imitation of consonant vowel combinations of increasing length and complexity.

Means of Communication

Emilio is a multimodal communicator who uses both oral language and an AAC system for the primary purpose of fulfilling basic wants and needs. He verbally communicates using a restricted set of one- and two-word phrases and he has an expressive vocabulary consisting of approximately 15 nouns and verbs collectively, all of which he produces with moderate intelligibility. There is a noted improvement in the accuracy and overall intelligibility of his speech following a verbal model. When asked a question or given a verbal command he frequently responds by repeating the last word of the prompt. For example, when asked, "Do you want to work for your iPad?" he would respond, "iPad." Educational staff believes Emilio's demonstration of echolalia is emerging functional communication and has hopes that an AAC system will facilitate and promote the expansion of verbal language.

AAC Use and Experience

Emilio has experience using an iPad with the Proloquo2go application. Emilio navigates through his AAC system to find preferred food items constructing three-word speech generated messages independently to communicate basic wants and needs. Emilio's AAC system consists of folders for preferred activities (4–5 icons) and food (i.e., fish crackers, juice, chips). Carrier phrases (e.g., "I want") were programmed as single icons.

Intervention

The intention of Emilio's participation in the intervention was multifold: (1) expand his language repertoire beyond the construct "noun" + "verb," (2) expand the purposes for which he communicates to include commenting, requesting social games, and sharing attention, and (3) support his expressive language (i.e., mean length of utterances, vocabulary) through the use of an AAC system. Intervention techniques consisted of shaping and fading/errorless teaching using a most intrusive (e.g., hand-over-hand) to least intrusive (e.g., gestural) prompting scale, modeling (both motor and verbal), and explaining expectations using simple language (e.g., "First we do this, then we can play on bouncy ball."). Emilio's tendency to elope in response to novel situations was averted by giving him an opportunity to request a break after participating in novel activities or newly introduced skills for a designated period of time that was gradually increased.

Description of AAC System

The biggest change to Emilio's communication system was the reorganization of his home page. His AAC system, an iPad with the Proloquo2go app, consisted of a main page comprised of 25 core vocabulary words and seven activity-specific folders that gave him access to fringe vocabulary related to various events (e.g. circle time, crafts, play activities). Table 7–2 provides a summary of Emilio's response to the intervention.

Response to Intervention

Emilio participated in a multitude of small and large group activities, including morning and afternoon circle, gross motor games (e.g. parachute, duck-duck-goose), and various crafts. He consistently used 3- to 4-word/symbol messages to communicate his wants and needs. He had to be broken of the habit of using a single icon to request a desired item. Emilio responded favorably when verbally prompted to "use more language." There was a noted increase in his use of verbal language to request wants and needs often pairing verbal language (e.g., 3- to 4-word sentences produced with improved intelligibility) with symbol use. Given a partial verbal prompt of "I," Emilio would verbalize "I want ___" using descriptive language (e.g. colors, size, quantity) to specify desired objects (e.g., "I want big ball." "I want more chase."). He also demonstrated growth in his ability to participate socially with peers for an extended period of time. Although he often shies away from novel people and situations, he has shown increased tolerance and comfort during such experiences.

Summary and Recommendations

It is recommended that intervention continue to focus on supporting Emilio in increasing his mean length of utterance, both verbally and symbolically, and expanding the grammatical complexity of his language. Continue to increase Emilio's tolerance of novel situations and new activities that provide him with an acceptable means to withdraw. Expand his use of language for various

Table 7–2. Summary of Emilio's Response to the Intervention

PLOPs	Intervention Targets	Progress
Emilio is dependent on both verbal and physical cues to transition his AAC system from one activity to the next (e.g., morning circle to his desk).	Emilio will independently transition his AAC system to different activities throughout his day with no more than 2 verbal cues per day (*Operational*).	Emilio independently transitioned his AAC system to all daily activities with no more than one verbal cue (e.g., "What do you need?") within a given day.
Emilio uses his communication system to request preferred objects, activities, and desired food items.	Given a model, Emilio will respond with a reciprocal comment (e.g. I have ___ or I see ___) related to the current activity on four out of five opportunities (*Social*).	Given a model and partial gestural prompt (i.e., pointing to his book) Emilio responded with a reciprocal comment related to the current activity using the symbols "have" and "see."
In response to a failed communication attempt Emilio will wait until he is prompted to repeat the message (e.g., "What do you want?").	Given a failed communication attempt, Emilio will use an appropriate gesture (e.g., tapping) to gain the attention of his communication partner and restate his message on four out of five opportunities (*Strategic*).	Emilio recognized when his communication attempts were missed and used a communication tap to gain his communication partner's attention prior to restating his messages on 100% of opportunities.
Emilio requests desired items using the sentence construct "I want" + preferred item.	Emilio will use a minimum of three different attributes (e.g. quantity, size, color) to request desired or necessary items within a structured activity (*Linguistic*).	Emilio used the descriptors: quantity (e.g. more), size (e.g. big/little), and colors to requests desired or necessary objects within a structured activity on three out of five opportunities.
Emilio uses primarily messages one- and two-symbols in length to express his wants/needs.	Emilio will use his AAC device to express messages at least three to four symbols in length (*Linguistic*).	Emilio used his AAC device to express messages at least 3 to 4 symbols in length.

other pragmatic functions that will expand his ability to interact with peers. As Emilio gains greater proficiency in his ability to use an AAC device for communication, consider exploring a language-based application (e.g., Speak for Yourself, Unity Language) and text-to- speech option. To facilitate ongoing AAC use and promote communication, consider the following recommendations and strategies:

- ◆ Expand Emilio's continued use of language for a range of communicative purposes by teaching him to utilize core vocabulary. Utilize a homepage with core vocabulary and specific folders for snack, circle time, craft, playtime, etc.
- ◆ Provide multiple opportunities throughout Emilio's day for him to utilize his device. For example, have him use his communication system to participate in class circle time and to request items during snack.
- ◆ Model use of Emilio's device throughout his day. For example, during craft activities pair oral language while pointing to corresponding symbols on Emilio's device.

CASE EXAMPLE #3: NOAH

Noah is a 3-year, 9-month-old male who qualifies for special education services under the eligibility of speech-language impaired. He presents with a history of developmental delays as a result of prenatal drug exposure. After delivery, Noah remained in the neonatal intensive care unit to give his body time to withdraw from the drug exposure. At the time of the intervention, Noah was enrolled in a non-categorical special education classroom (SDC) preschool. In addition to his SDC placement, Noah received speech and language intervention services that were provided through the school district, along with occupational and physical therapies. His IEP goals that related to speech and language skills were written to expand single word labeling, imitation of 2- to 3-word sentences, and following one-step activity related directions.

Means of Communication

Noah could best be described as both an intentional and non-intentional communicator. As a multimodal communicator, he uses symbolic (i.e., gestures, manual signs, verbal approximations, and emerging symbol use) and non-symbolic (behaviors) forms of communication to express basic wants and needs, as well as to protest. Receptive language skills are reported as a relative strength in comparison to his expressive language abilities. Noah demonstrates understanding of basic commands and requests (e.g., let's go, come here, go there, time to play, snack time) and recognizes pictorial symbols (e.g., colored line drawings). He primarily uses 1- to 2-word phrases and rote word phrases (e.g., such as "more, I want ____, please, all done, yes, no, and yeah"). During baseline testing, Noah receptively identified a variety of Picture Communication Symbols (PCS™) symbols including: nouns (ball, car, shoe, cookies, juice, book, banana, dog, baby, mom, bedroom, home, and square), verbs (sleep, eat, wash, drink, read, ride, and play), adjectives (wet, big, small, middle, square, tall, and first), and prepositions (on, under, in, and in front of).

AAC Use and Experience

Prior to the intervention, Noah had no prior experience with any type of formal AAC system, either low tech or high tech. He had learned a few manual signs (e.g., "more" and "want") but was only using them during snack.

Intervention

The overarching goal of Noah's participation in the intervention was to increase his communicative intent, increase his overall engagement and compliance to adult-directed activities with peers, and expand his expressive language skills either verbally or through the use of an AAC system. His communication guide modeled how to use his communication system by pointing to the symbols as she spoke, and directing Noah's finger to select symbols to create messages. Due to Noah's young age and overall level of functioning relative to other students enrolled in the program, he was given frequent "breaks" involving more active types (e.g., bubbles, balloon play) of interactions in which communication was equally targeted. It was difficult for Noah to sustain his attention for an extended period of time in teacher-directed activities requiring students to remain seated for a lengthy period of time. Having a place in the room where he could go to interact with his communication guide without interrupting the entire group proved extremely beneficial. To improve Noah's ability to attend to adult-directed activities for increasing periods of time, a token board behavior management system was implemented. Noah earned tokens for staying on task and participating in large group activities. Once he earned five tokens, he earned a preferred reinforcement. Although food (e.g., fish crackers) was used as a quick reinforcer to get him back to being engaged in the current activity, he also requested more social types of reinforcers (e.g., playing go and stop with balloon). His communication guide routinely expanded on his utterances and used self-talk (e.g., "Oh, you asked me for peanut butter, so here is your peanut butter." "You said go, so here I go!") to enrich his language experiences. Consistency was critical for his success. His communication guide interpreted his symbol use, literally responding to his communication attempts even knowing that was not necessarily his intentions. He learned quickly to make adjustments in his messages to achieve his desired outcomes. A prompting hierarchy (e.g., verbal cue, facial expressions, pausing) was constantly in practice and only using full models or hand-over-hand modeling when he was not responding or responding incorrectly.

Description of Communication System

A no-tech flipbook design communication system was developed for Noah. Noah's AAC system consisted of a primary core page comprised of 40 core vocabulary words and strips of activity specific fringe words that were spiral bound to the top of the primary core page. This arrangement gave Noah routine access to core vocabulary and he could flip to the activity-related fringe strips. There were, on average, seven symbols per each category/activity-based fringe strip (e.g., people, craft-supplies, food items, and utensils). The construction of the Noah's communication book allowed him to easily navigate through the strips to find related fringe words. A cover was added and a handle constructed out of rope and beads that made the entire system durable, light, and easily portable. Table 7–3 provides a list of the core vocabulary words that were available to Noah. Table 7–4 provides the specific skills that were targeted during the intervention, including Noah's baseline performance related to these specific targets and his progress.

Table 7–3. Noah's Core Vocabulary Set

Pronouns	Verbs	Prepositions	Adjectives	Questions	Misc.
I	do	on	little	what	here
you	play	off	big	who	don't
my	put	out	happy	where	that
your	like	in	angry		more
everybody	help	up	sad		all done
it	want				
	turn				
	make				
	stop				
	go				
	read				
	look				
	open				
	have				
	turn				
	close				

Table 7–4. Summary of Noah's Response to the Intervention

PLOPs	Intervention Targets	Progress
Noah's uses single words and a restricted set of 2- to 3-word utterances to request preferred food items and objects (e.g., "more," "I want ___," "please," "all done," "yes," "no," and "yeah"). He uses the sentence construct pronoun + noun, with an occasional addition of a verb (e.g., "I <u>want</u> juice" and "more juice").	Given a communication system consisting of both core vocabulary and fringe words, Noah will expand his sentence structure to include pronoun + verb + object to communicate during structured activities (*Linguistic*).	Noah expanded his sentence constructions to include "pronoun + verb + object" (e.g., I push it, You do it) and action-direction (e.g., go up, go, down, you go) structures. Given a verbal and aided model Noah imitated 3- to 4-word/symbol utterances.
Noah is able to identify a variety of symbols including nouns, verbs, adjectives, and prepositions.	Given a field of 15 to 20 symbols, Noah will demonstrate understanding and use of eight new core vocabulary words/symbols (*Linguistic*).	Given a field of 28 symbols, Noah demonstrated understanding and use of 14 new core vocabulary symbols.
Noah is able to retrieve his lunch bag at snack time given several verbal prompts.	Noah will independently transition his communication notebook between activities or locations, over at least two structured activities, over two consecutive days, as measured by the clinician (*Operational*).	Noah independently transitioned his communication board three to four times each day.
Noah currently communicates to fulfill his basic wants and needs.	Noah will expand the purposes for which he communicates by using his communication system for at least two different purposes other than requesting preferred food items and objects, over two consecutive days, as measured by the clinician (*Social*).	Noah used communication to direct the behavior of another person (e.g., "You go"), initiate a social interaction (e.g., saying "hello/goodbye"), seek attention of a peer or familiar adult, and comment about personal actions. Noah is learning to communicate to share information with hand-over-hand modeling,

continues

Table 7–4. *continued*

PLOPs	Intervention Targets	Progress
Noah currently participates during reading and singing by watching others, use of non-symbolic behaviors, and occasional verbal approximations.	Given a book or song with a repetitive phrase or word, Noah will participate in the reading/ singing of the book/ song by either vocalizing the predictable word or phrase and/or selecting the appropriate symbol on his communication system (*Social*).	Given a book or song with a repetitive phrase or word, Noah independently participated in the reading/singing of the book/song by either vocalizing the predictable word or phrase and/ or selecting the appropriate symbol on his communication board.
When Noah's communication attempts are misunderstood or he does not get the response he desires, he will respond by verbally protesting (e.g., "no or more") and/or displaying unacceptable behaviors (e.g., tantrum or eloping).	Given a failed communication attempt, Noah will gain the attention of his communication partner via gesture or vocalization and repeat his message (*Strategic*).	When his communication partner failed to respond to his communication attempts Noah gained her attention by tapping her on the arm and with prompting to his communication board he repeated his message.
Noah can currently identify pictorial symbols in his direct view.	During a structured activity, Noah will turn pages on his communication board to find a desired symbol that is out of view (*Strategic*).	During a structured activity, Noah navigated through the pages on his communication board to find desired and necessary symbols.

Response to Intervention

During camp, Noah enjoyed participating in group songs, dance, shared readings, and playing with his peers. In his regular classroom, participation in these types of activities was often difficult or met with resistance. Noah made significant progress over the course of the intense intervention. Not only did he expand his knowledge and use of symbols to include core vocabulary, but he increased the length of his messages and expanded his sentence structures. Post intervention, Noah increased his expressive vocabulary and mean length of utterance, by using two to three core and fringe vocabulary words in the sentence construction of pronoun + verb + noun. Noah demonstrated an increased understanding of both transparent (easily recognizable) and opaque (not easily recognizable) core vocabulary words on his communication board, and independently navigated through his communication system to search for desired fringe words that were not in his current view. He enjoyed matching words spoken by his communication guide with corresponding symbols represented on his communication system. Noah independently transitioned his communication system, benefitting from occasional verbal (e.g., "What do you need?") or visual cues (e.g., point to his communication system, giving him a look of "are you forgetting something"), all of which were continually faded until the last day when he demonstrated increased independence in transitioning his communication system from one activity to another. He expanded the purposes for which he communicated to include directing the behavior of another person for mutual enjoyment, sharing information, initiating social interactions, and participating in group activities. Noah demonstrated the ability to repair communication breakdowns with a partner by saying "no" and directly selecting the symbols that were available to him. He quickly learned that symbols correspond with verbal language and was motivated to navigate through his communication board independently.

Suggestions and Recommendations

Noah's receptive language continues to be strength in comparison to his expressive language skills. Therefore continued use of an AAC system is critical to bridge this gap. It is recommended that he continue to use his communication system in the classroom and expand its use to home not only for the purposes of communicating, but for the purposes of supporting his expressive language skills as well. As Noah demonstrates continued benefit from using his communication system to communicate and facilitate production of oral language, the IEP team may want to explore a more sophisticated type of communication system that would give him greater access to an expanding vocabulary set. He would also benefit from the following recommendations.

- ◆ Use Noah's AAC system to expand on his communication attempts. For example, if he says "more," verbally model "more what?" while simultaneously pointing to corresponding pictures in his communication book.
- ◆ Teach Noah to recognize different facial expressions through the use of his communication book (e.g., a fringe strip consisting of emotions: happy, sad, angry, and tired). Periodically, throughout his day, help him identify emotions of self and others, including modeling how to use his communication book to express emotions (e.g., simultaneously saying "I am hungry, you hungry?" while pointing to corresponding pictures on his communication book).

◆ Model communication for purposes of sharing information. For example, when reading a book, ask questions related to the story giving Noah an opportunity to comment on characters' actions:

> COMMUNICATION GUIDE: "What did it (rabbit) do?"
>
> NOAH: "Go fast."
>
> COMMUNICATION GUIDE: "Do you like this story?"
>
> NOAH: "Yes, I like it!"
>
> *Always remembering to pair oral language models with picture symbols.

◆ Scaffold opportunities for Noah to use his communication book throughout the day and across multiple activities and environments (both at home and at school).

◆ Model communication opportunities. Prompt Noah to use his communication book when you observe a communication opportunity (e.g., When you observe Noah struggling to open a container. You respond by providing him with the verbal prompt and model, "Your language is, 'I want help'").

◆ Establish regular communication between the school speech-language pathologist and parent/caregiver to encourage consistency of intervention techniques and strategies.

CASE EXAMPLE #4: NATALIA

Natalia is a 15-year-old female who qualifies for special education services with a primary eligibility of autism and a secondary eligibility of cognitive impairment. At the time of the intervention Natalia was enrolled in a self-contained special education classroom for five of her seven classes. With the support of an instructional aide, she was mainstreamed for physical education and one elective course (e.g., art, music). Natalia participated in a daily communication class, and support staff worked to scaffold communication opportunities throughout her day.

Means of Communication

Natalia's primary means of communication is through vocalizations. Expressive communication is characterized by one-word utterances spoken in a low volume at a fast rate. She will vocalize to indicate discomfort or need to use the restroom, to gain someone's attention, and to indicate displeasure with the current activity or expectation.

AAC Use and Experience

Natalia has been exposed to a myriad of AAC interventions over the course of her education, including a communication notebook and low-tech communication systems (e.g., Go Talk 20) with varying success. Her most recent communication notebook was a two-inch, three-ring binder filled with over 50 one-inch laminated picture icons adhered to pages with Velcro. Along with key phrases (e.g., I want, I want break, I need bathroom), pictured items included preferred food items and activities, class subjects, and relevant school supplies. Natalia was recently introduced to the Speak for Yourself app loaded on the iPad.

Intervention

The purpose of Natalia's participation in the two-week intervention pro-gram was to provide her with an intensive block of intervention to firmly establish her AAC skills and facilitate her AAC use across environment and activities. Since being introduced to the iPad with the Speak for Yourself app, Natalia demonstrates interest in using her AAC system to communicate. She learns new skills following initial models but because skills are not firmly established, she frequently has to re-learn previously taught skills when they are reintroduced three days to a week later. Table 7–5 provides the specific skills that were targeted during the intervention, including Natalia's baseline performance related to these specific targets and her progress.

Description of Communication System:

Natalia uses an iPad 2 with the communication app Speak for Yourself.

Response to Intervention

Natalia made significant gains through her participation in the two-week intense intervention program. In addition to making progress toward her goals in all four competency areas, she increased her ability to attend to adult-directed activities and increased her social awareness and interest in peers. Upon the conclusion of the intervention program, she was independently greeting her communication guide by name, as well as her peers. She was emerging in her use of four- and five-symbols messages, expanding the purpose for which she communicated beyond requesting preferred food items, objects, and activities, and fulfilling immediate needs.

Table 7–5. Summary of Natalia's Response to the Intervention

PLOPs	Intervention Targets	Progress
Following a verbal prompt, Natalia will use the sentence construction "I want + (preferred food item or activity) + please with her iPad.	Natalia will use four-symbol message using at least three different sentence constructions (*Linguistic*).	Using her iPad, Natalia consistently constructed four and occasionally five-symbol messages consisting of actors (i.e., I, you), actions (e.g., put, take, go), objects, attributes (e.g., color, quantity, size), and locations (i.e., in, there, here).
Natalia identifies a variety of picture icons specific to preferred food items and activities, classroom materials, and locations (e.g., home, restaurant).	Natalia will demonstrate knowledge and use of 15 new core vocabulary words and five activity related fringe words (*Linguistic*).	Natalia expanded her understanding and use of 20 new core vocabulary words (e.g., put, on, need, my, turn, go, no, see, play) and 10 new fringe words (e.g., stickers, tape, desk).
In response to a greeting posed by a peer and a prompt to say, "Hi," Natalia will imitate "Hi" looking at the ground unless prompted to look at the person.	Given a familiar routine and a prompt to use her device, Natalia will independently greet a peer or familiar adult using her device (*Social*).	Within the morning routine of greeting peers and given a greeting by a peer followed by an expectant delay, Natalia used her communication system to greet a peer.
Natalia vocalizes and expresses single words to request and protest without directing her communication attempts to any specific person. When her communication attempts are not recognized, she often becomes visibly upset.	Given a failed communication attempt, Natalia will gain her communication partner's attention ether by vocalizing and/or tapping them on the arm, establishing eye contact, and then redelivering her message (*Strategic*).	After multiple opportunities to practice this skill that was initially introduced with hand-over-hand modeling and then with less obtrusive prompts (i.e., gestural prompt to wait paired with an expectant delay) Natalia was learning to use this strategy to initiate and to redeliver a missed message by the conclusion of the intervention.
Natalia currently uses the pictures icons available to her on her front page.	Given a communication opportunity, Natalia will navigate through her communication system to find desired icons (*Operational*).	Natalia can access icons on her first page, select the appropriate folder to find relevant icons to routine-based activities, and return to her home page independently.

Suggestions and Recommendations

In order to facilitate her ongoing acquisition of new skills and continued establishment of newly acquired skills, the following recommendations should be considered:

◆ Create communication opportunities for her throughout her day. For example, when facilitating an activity, purposefully omit key steps or necessary materials prompting her to direct you "to fix" what is left out or missing.
◆ Expand on her communication attempts by modeling on her device how to expand her content or length of her messages.
◆ Model more complex forms of language.
◆ Provide her with opportunities to recognizing missed messages and redelivering those messages.

CASE EXAMPLE #5: ETHAN

Ethan is a 9-year, 2-month-old male who presents with a primary diagnosis of intellectual disability and a secondary diagnosis of autism. At the time of the intervention, he was enrolled in a non-categorical 4th grade special day class (SDC). In addition to his SDC placement, he concurrently received speech and language services to address delays in the areas of expressive and receptive language skills, compounded by a diagnosis of severe apraxia of speech. His IEP goals related to speech and language skills were written to improve his articulation in producing /f, k, g/ in all positions of words, answer "Wh" questions, use language to request, comment, and retell short stories.

Means of Communication

Ethan's primary means of communication prior to the onset of the intervention was oral communication augmented through gestures, facial expressions, and eye gaze. His overall speech intelligibility was understood 20 to 25% of the time, given a known context ,and less than 15% given an unfamiliar context. Expressive language was characterized by 2- to 4-word utterance approximations. He used simple rote sentences (e.g., I want ___, My turn, No, my ___) when communicating and seeking social interactions with peers. Ethan's primary strategies for initiating conversations and social interactions with peers consisted of vocalizing, tapping a peer's arm or shoulder, or bringing an object of interest to share with a peer. When Ethan encountered a communication barrier (e.g., needing help to open his snack), he often had difficulty communicating his needs (e.g., I need help, please) and he would frequently revert to physical behaviors (e.g., grabbing a person's arm to request assistance, throwing the object away, pushing a friend away instead of telling them to "stop"). A token system was used during tasks to support Ethan in having a "good attitude" and demonstrating positive behavior toward finishing a task and listening to the teacher.

AAC Use and Experience

Ethan's classroom teacher recently introduced a communication system based on picture exchange. Although this communication system was not used consistently, Ethan recognized familiar and concrete pictures and symbols, and understood that putting two or more symbols together created a meaning and a response from his communication partner. He used this system primarily for the purposes of requesting food items and preferred reinforcers.

Intervention

The overarching goal of Ethan's participation in the intensive intervention was to expand his verbal communication skills and to help him learn strategies to compensate in the event of a communication breakdown. Ethan's communication system was designed with several purposes in mind. Although Ethan readily imitated familiar two-word phrases on the first attempt, he struggled to imitate novel or less familiar phrases or messages greater than two words in length. Pairing oral verbal models with visual symbols gave Ethan the auditory input and visual cues he needed to produce longer, more complex messages. Additionally Ethan's communication system allowed his communication guide to pair her verbal models with visual support, not only demonstrating to him how to use his system in real time, but providing him with the visual support he needed to improve his ability to comprehend more complex language. Finally, Ethan's communication system gave him an additional means to clarify his messages when his communication attempts were not understood.

Description of Communication System

Ethan's communication system, which was refined over the first two days of the program, consisted of a communication board comprised of 63 core vocabulary words, with a space for activity-specific fringe vocabulary to be changed out as needed. Table 7–6 provides a list of the core vocabulary words that were available to Ethan. These words were selected based on Ethan's needs and the words his communication guide needed available to model more complex forms of language relevant to the various tasks. Table 7–7 provides the specific skills that were targeted during intervention, including Ethan's baseline performance related to these specific targets and his progress.

Table 7–6. Ethan's Core Vocabulary Set

Pronouns	Verbs	Prepositions	Adjectives	Questions	Misc.
I	do	to	little	why	here
you	can	next	big	what	there
me	i	with	happy	who	this
my	like	inside	mad	where	that
	help	on	sad	how	don't
	want	off	awesome		no
	put	out	cool		yes
	turn	in			that
	make	up			more
	get	down			some
	stop	over			again
	go				
	come				
	feel				
	eat				
	drink				
	look				
	please				
	open				
	need				
	have				
	give				
	read				

Response to Intervention

Ethan responded positively to locating, using, and accessing his communication board to request, clarify, or ask questions. He learned new words quickly, given an initial model provided by his communication guide, he manipulated core vocabulary with fringe vocabulary to construct an expanded range of sentence structures, and he was emerging in his ability to formulate and express four- to six-word sentences using picture symbols. Ethan's communicative intent extended beyond requesting preferred objects to include

Table 7–7. Summary of Ethan's Response to the Intervention

PLOPs	Intervention Targets	Progress
Ethan imitates 2-word phrases with 90% accuracy. He uses phrases and sentences 2 to 6 words in length but his communication partners can only understand up to 2 words due to his apraxia.	Ethan will respond using three- to four-word sentences within a structured activity, given a verbal prompt (e.g. what materials do you need?) and the visual support of his communication board (*Linguistic*).	Ethan has made great progress in this area. He consistently used and imitated three- to four-word sentences (e.g., "Come on Jacob," "Hey, it my turn"), and up to five- to six-word symbol/word sentences with the support of his communication board (e.g., "I want some more fish please).
When prompted to use his communication board, Ethan has the choice to use statements to fulfill immediate desires and needs (e.g., "I want art area, I want playground").	Ethan will demonstrate use of five new different types of sentences (e.g., statements, exclamations, requests, or questions) with familiar adults or peers during structured activities (*Linguistic*).	Ethan used five types of sentences, including statements and requests. Given the opportunity to ask a question (e.g., clinician prompts him to ask a question by saying, "Ask me"), Ethan formulated simple sentences and questions (e.g., "Can I have ___?" "Who turn?" "Do you want ___?").
Ethan uses his communication board when prompted by his teacher and paraprofessionals.	Ethan will independently locate, access, and use his communication board during structured activities and peer interactions in the classroom (*Operational*).	Ethan consistently and independently located, accessed, and used his communication board with ease. He enjoyed having his communication board close by to take advantage of the opportunities to express, ask, or share ideas with his peers.
Ethan seeks out social interactions with his peers in the classroom by taking objects or toys from his peers. On the playground, he initiates social interactions by tapping his friends on the shoulder and then running away to initiate a game of tag.	Given a communication breakdown, Ethan will respond to his communication partner's request for clarification by using his communication board to clarify his message (*Strategic*).	When given the opportunity to initiate conversations with others, Ethan independently used his communication board after the clinician modeled the question or sentence 2 to 3 times (e.g., "Do you want paint?" "I like that").

asking questions and making comments and statements. Likewise, the use of his communication board gave him a strategy to clarify the meaning of his messages in the event of a communication breakdown. He continued to benefit from occasional reminders to look at his communication board as he spoke because his verbal output was not always consistent with symbols he was pointing to (e.g., He says, "I want water," but points to the "give" symbol instead of the "want" symbol). This inaccuracy may be the result of too much stimuli in the classroom (e.g., noise, movement of bodies, talking) or fatigue. Overall, Ethan has made great progress in his communication skills with the support of his board.

Suggestions and Recommendations

The progress Ethan demonstrated during the two-week intervention supports his use of a communication board to support his communicative intents and verbal output. In order to continue his successes in using an assistive and augmentative communication (AAC) notebook, recommendations include:

◆ Integrate and support his continued use of his communication board in classroom activities and during communication breakdowns.
◆ Provide Ethan with constant access to core vocabulary and fringe vocabulary that may change accordingly to the activity at hand.
◆ Pair verbal language models with picture symbols consistently to further expand his language use and the length of his utterances while demonstrating to him how he can use communication throughout his day.
◆ Encourage practice and use of his communication board (e.g., "I want some more") to increase his familiarity of the board and ultimately automaticity with knowing the location of the icons.

CASE EXAMPLE #6: AARON

Aaron, a 5-year, 1-month-old male, presents with a medical diagnosis of cerebral palsy. Aaron is non-ambulatory and requires assistance for loco-motion (e.g., a manual wheelchair) and toileting (e.g., aided assistance). He qualifies for special education services with a primary eligibility of orthopedic impairment and a secondary eligibility of speech-language impairment. He is enrolled in a non-categorical preschool special day class but will be transition-ing into a general education classroom beginning in the fall for kindergarten. He receives 60 minutes of speech and language intervention services through the school district to address goals for improving breath support, increas-ing loudness of speech, improving syntax, and implementing conversational repair strategies. He receives occupational and physical therapies through the state's children services. He can independently feed himself by balancing food on his right hand using an adaptive utensil. Aaron's oral motor functioning is severely compromised due to a diagnosis of moderate-to-severe dysarthria, which is characterized by drooling, weak oral musculature, and slurred speech. Vocal quality is weak and strained due to decreased breath support.

Means of Communication

Aaron primarily communicates through oral communication. His overall speech intelligibility and ability to produce an age-appropriate utterance length is compromised by his dysarthria and weak respiratory support. Aaron augments his speech with non-symbolic forms of communication such as vocalizations, facial expressions, head movements, and eye gaze. Due to decreased breath support, Aaron is only capable of producing two- to three-word utterances and phrases. Aaron will readily repeat phrases using a louder voice when requested to do so. When Aaron is unable to communicate, he withdraws from conversations and ceases making communication attempts. Aaron is motivated to communicate with peers and adults. He will initiate communication and social interactions using eye gaze and facial gestures. He actively participates in conversations and responds to questions. Responses frequently consist of facial expressions, head movements, and shifts in eye gaze. Aaron will offer verbal responses when requested and/or prompted to do so.

AAC Experience and Use

Prior to the implementation of the intervention program, Aaron was evaluated for an AAC system. The AAC intervention served as part of the trial period. In order for Aaron's communication device to be funded through either his medical insurance or Medi-Cal, he needed to demonstrate the ability to use his communication system for a wide range of communicative purposes, including relaying needs related to adaptive skills.

Intervention

The primary purpose for Aaron's participation in the two-week intervention was to provide him with an intensive block of intervention focused on teaching him how to use his AAC system. Additionally, it provided an opportunity for his instructional assistant, who had limited experience in area of AAC, to gain valuable hands-on-opportunities programming his system and facilitating Aaron's use of his device. This was a critical piece in successfully transitioning Aaron from a self-contained SDC preschool to being fully integrated into a general education kindergarten.

Description of Communication System

Aaron used the Accent 800, preloaded with the Unity language system from PRC. The Unity language system uses a small set of recognizable picture icons that, when combined in short sequences, produces words, phrases, and sentences. The first screen is comprised of core words that are strategically organized to facilitate language use. The Accent 800 is a small, lightweight portable device. Aaron's device was either situated on the tray of his wheelchair or in his lap. With a key guard, Aaron used the knuckle of his index finger to directly access picture icons from a field of 32 icons. Table 7–8 provides the specific skills that were targeted during the intervention, including Aaron's baseline performance related to these specific targets, and his progress.

Response to Intervention

Aaron made significant gains during the two-week intervention program. He quickly demonstrated an understanding with regards to navigating Unity language software, and accessing the Accent 800. Initially, Aaron needed a single visual model to locate high frequency and high interest vocabulary on the device prior to locating vocabulary independently. He would remember the location of preferred icons from day-to-day (e.g., numerals). Aaron learned to independently modify his language output and increase efficiency by restricting the number of hits required to produce a phrase. For instance, instead of using four hits to say, "thank you," he would use "thanks," which only required two hits. Aaron was able to access the device by physically adjusting the proximity of the device to maximize his ability to hit target icons using his left and right knuckles. Throughout camp, Aaron was highly motivated and enthusiastic about using his device, especially when emphasizing a desire to navigate the system independently (e.g., "I want to do it."). Aaron is capable of locating desired vocabulary after a single demonstration. He continues to require verbal prompting to produce more complex and syntactically correct phrases, typically preferring to use one- to two-word phrases. Aaron uses multimodal forms of communication by combining oral communication with device-based communication. He will resolve communication breakdowns using his device to clarify a statement by repeating and/ or restating a phrase. Aaron is able to identify when icons were hit in error and will independently clear the screen prior to making a second attempt at creating a desired phrase. With support, Aaron is capable of constructing four- to five-word phrases. His verbalizations continue to be characterized by weak voicing and moderate to severe dysarthria. Ultimately, Aaron has demonstrated the language, cognitive, motor, and social skills necessary to achieve his functional communication goals using an augmentative communication device.

Table 7–8. Summary of Aaron's Response to the Intervention

PLOPs	Intervention Targets	Progress
Aaron uses primarily single word responses and 2-to 3-word phrases when prompted to use more language. He is primarily a responder, but will initiate interactions using non-verbal means. He has no prior AAC experience.	Aaron will independently navigate through his AAC device to locate high frequency and activity specific fringe vocabulary (*Operational*).	Aaron independently located high frequency core vocabulary words and activity specific fringe vocabulary words on his AAC device.
Based on the AAC assessment, Aaron can select a subject and object from a given field of picture symbols to produce a message, but he does not currently include verbs.	Aaron will use a language-based software program to request, comment, or label constructing three symbol messages (subject-verb-object) within a concrete activity/routine (e.g., girl eat cookie), with one verbal and/or visual prompt. (*Linguistic*)	Aaron consistently created three symbol messages (subject-verb-object) within familiar activities and routines when provided with the verbal prompt, "Use more language," to expand the complexity of his messages.
Aaron uses primarily single word responses and 2- to 3-word phrases when prompted to use more language. He is primarily a responder but will initiate interactions using non-verbal means. He uses non-symbolic behavioral forms of communication (e.g., facial grimaces, eye contact).	Aaron will engage in no fewer than three conversational turns, including conversation starters, with familiar adults or peers using a language-based software program. (*Social*)	Aaron used his device to engage in up to two conversational turns, when provided with a verbal prompt to maintain communication using his device during social exchanges.
Aaron will withdraw from conversations and communicative attempts when communication breakdowns occur.	Given a communication breakdown that occurs when making a device-based request, Aaron will modify and/or repeat a target phrase until his listener responds. (*Strategic*)	Aaron attempted to resolve communication breakdowns when prompted to use his device as a method of rephrasing an unclear verbal request. He also repeated a word or phrase when the listener does not provide a desired response.

Suggestions and Recommendations

Aaron may benefit from the following strategies to further develop his communication competence with his communication device:

◆ Use his communication device on a daily basis. The language systems being considered for Aaron (e.g., TouchChat w/Word Power, Speak for Yourself) are complex and require consistency of use, similar to learning a second language. Without continued exposure and use, Aaron will not be able to retain the skills necessary to effectively and efficiently operate his communication system.

◆ Provide Aaron with communication opportunities. Refrain from addressing Aaron using yes/no questions, which restrict his language output. Provide him with opportunities to respond to open-ended questions and encourage social engagement among peers and adults, including initiating social interactions.

◆ Encourage Aaron to be a multimodal communicator. Aaron is fully capable of producing complex language using both verbalizations and a communication device. Aaron should continue to incorporate verbalizations, vocalizations, gestures, eye-gaze, and facial expressions in conjunction with a speech-generating device, as a total augmentative communication approach.

◆ Require the use of speaking with a strong voice. Impaired respiration results in weakened voicing, which contributes to decreased intelligibility. Aaron will attempt to restate unclear phrases when prompted to take a deep breath and use a "strong voice." Gentle tactile compression on Aaron's rib cage can assist with providing more respiratory support for voicing.

◆ Continue to explore device access. Experiment with various devices to determine which will provide Aaron with the greatest amount of access (e.g., the iPad versus the Accent 800). It is essential that a device support overall efficiency, so as not to inhibit his ability to communicate fluently with others.

CASE EXAMPLE #7: MAGGIE

Maggie is a 5-year, 4-month-old female who qualifies for special education services under the eligibility of "autistic-like characteristics" and "speech/language impairment." At the time of the intervention, she was enrolled in a preschool special day class specifically designed for students with autism. She also received speech-language and occupational therapies. Speech-language goals were written to increase understanding of prepositions (i.e., in, on, off, out), increase rate of initiation for the purposes of fulfilling basic desires, and imitating sentences of increasing length and complexity.

Means of Communication

As a multimodal communicator, Maggie uses oral language paired with a picture exchange communication system for the purposes of requesting. Verbal communication is characterized by 1- to 2-word utterances that she uses to fulfill basic wants and needs and to request preferred reinforcers. Maggie follows a variety of two-step routine based directives, as well as commands constructed of one noun and one verb (e.g., baby eat, dad go, eat apple). Maggie imitates sentence up to four words in length containing the following syntactic structures and morphological markers: auxiliary form of the verb "to be," present progressive, prepositions "in" and "on," early attributes, and possessives "my" and "your."

Baseline measures indicated she receptively identifies a variety of PCS™ symbols on a board consisting of 32 icons. Although she demonstrates the ability to expressively label individual pictures, she struggles to demonstrate her knowledge when asked to point to a specific picture on command (e.g., show me or point to . . .). Maggie also demonstrates difficulty attending to structured tasks for extended periods of time, as well as maintaining eye contact with communication partners.

AAC Use and Experience

Maggie's AAC experience consisted of using a picture exchange communication book comprised of the phrase "I want" and pictures and symbols of preferred food items and objects. She uses her communication book primarily during snack.

Intervention

The goals of Maggie's participation in the intensive two-week intervention were to expand her communication ability. Prior to the intervention, she used her communication system primarily for the purposes of fulfilling basic needs and immediate wants, and she was heavily dependent on direction from others to initiate her interaction even in the presence of a communication temptation.

Description of Communication System

Throughout camp, Maggie used a communication board consisting of 26 core vocabulary with strips of fringe vocabulary symbols located above the core board. Fringe words could be flipped and included everyday camp vocabulary words for activities, such as making lemonade, snack time, and preferred toys. Her communication guide also included a strip of commenting picture symbols that included words such as "see," "taste," "feel," and "yummy." Her book also included communication boards specific to songs and books that were used every day. Table 7–9 provides a summary of Maggie's response to the intervention.

Response to Intervention

Since AAC Camp began, Maggie has made significant progress in her verbal communication. Maggie has been requesting with more independence and creating longer utterances as well. She also creates utterances for the purpose of commenting either spontaneously or with clinician prompting. For example, she would spontaneously use the phrase "I see ____." throughout a camp day or would complete a phrase started by the clinician. She worked hard when her attention was gained and learned new language quickly when given a verbal model. She enjoyed the songs and books that were sung and read every day at camp and verbalized the accompanying words independently. Maggie was also able to recognize a variety of picture communication symbols independently.

Suggestions and Recommendations

The following are a few strategies to further support Maggie's acquisition of communication:

◆ Expand on Maggie's communication: When Maggie communicates using single words or short utterances, her communication guide can model more language while pointing to picture symbols on his communication book. For example, if she verbally says "mouse," respond, "Yes, I see a blue mouse," simultaneously pointing to corresponding symbols. This aided language modeling strategy will provide her with both a visual and verbal expansion of her original utterance.

◆ Use visual communication symbols to support her communication: Because Maggie benefits from visual supports, it will be helpful to model language use on her communication board by pointing to the appropriate symbols. For example, if you are introducing new language to her, point to the appropriate symbols on her communication board as you say each word slowly. You could also take her hand and help her point to each symbol as you are saying the utterance so she has a visual model as well as a verbal model.

Table 7–9. Summary of Maggie's Response to the Intervention

PLOPs	Intervention Targets	Progress
Maggie primarily uses single or two-word utterances following a verbal model or given a visual referent and prompt to communicate for the purposes of requesting preferred objects and activities.	Maggie will independently use her communication board to create utterances of at least three symbols in length, 15 times a day during classroom activities as measured by clinician data (*Linguistic*).	Maggie produced utterances 3 to 4 words in length for requesting purposes, approximately 20 times throughout the day either independently or with minimal prompting by her communication guide. She also produced utterances of 2 to 3 words in length for the purposes of commenting approximately 15 times throughout her day with prompting to use her book.
Maggie demonstrates understanding of a wide range of picture icons by receptively pointing to them on request.	Maggie will independently use her index finger to access relevant picture symbols on her communication board when given a field of 26 symbols during an activity with 80% accuracy as measured by clinician data (*Operational*).	Maggie accessed a variety of symbols when requesting or commenting during camp-themed activities given a communication board consisting of 26 core vocabulary symbols. Maggie independently accessed her preferred fringe words (e.g., cookies) with 90% accuracy.
Maggie demonstrates difficulty maintaining eye contact with other individuals and has trouble focusing on identified task.	Maggie will establish eye contact when commenting to a peer or familiar adult during structured activities (*Social*).	When asked to greet another peer/counselor, Maggie established eye contact in approximately 4 out of 5 opportunities with minimal prompting (e.g., expectant delay). Eye contact significantly improved when she tapped her communication partner on the shoulder in order to gain his or her attention.

continues

Table 7–9. *continued*

PLOPs	Intervention Targets	Progress
Maggie demonstrates difficulty directing her messages towards specific individuals when communicating. She often requests without using eye contact and taps on the picture symbol she is referring to. She also has difficulty establishing and maintaining joint attention.	Maggie will independently gain the attention of a peer/familiar adult by tapping him/her on the arm when he needs assistance or wants to communicate in 4 out of 5 opportunities as measured by clinician data (*Strategic*).	Maggie gained the attention of her communication guide by tapping her on the shoulder when she wanted to communicate or needed help approximately 10 times during snack, establishing eye contact 70% of the time. She began generalizing this tapping strategy to other activities, as well as to other adults and peers.

It would also be beneficial to provide visual supports in a variety of communication opportunities to help support Maggie's language understanding. For example, she benefited from picture schedules and visual supports for songs/books during camp.

◆ Maintain eye contact: To improve Maggie's ability to maintain eye contact with others, she was taught how to gain another person's attention by tapping someone on the shoulder. This strategy also improved her ability to maintain eye contact with her communication partner so it is suggested that this strategy be implemented in other environments. The communication partner should initially face away from Maggie when she is trying to communicate or she wants a preferred item that he/she has. This creates an opportunity for Maggie to gain his/her attention and to establish eye contact.

◆ Create communication opportunities: It is important to generalize Maggie's commenting abilities to other environments and people. For example, if a familiar individual is approaching, you can point to the person and say, "Look! I see ____ coming. Let's say hi to her." You can have her repeat, "I see ____." Then you can go over to the individual and have Maggie say, "Hi ____." This strategy will help to generalize phrases specific to commenting and greetings to other environments and people.

CASE EXAMPLE #8: WYATT

Wyatt, a 12-year, 10-month-old male, presents with a primary eligibility of autism and a secondary diagnosis of intellectual disability. He receives all academic instruction in self-contained special education classes. In addition to specialized academic instruction, he receives speech and language therapy, occupational therapy, adapted physical education, assistive technology services, and intensive behavioral services.

Means of Communication

Wyatt currently communicates utilizing an iPad programmed with the Speak For Yourself app, an application that includes a large core and fringe vocabulary set with synthesized speech output. Wyatt is able to use his iPad functionally throughout his day during both structured and unstructured activities. During structured activities, Wyatt can answer simple yes/no questions. During unstructured activities, he can request preferred food items, objects and activities. Receptively, Wyatt follows routine-based multistep directions. Expressively, he responds to novel topics and participates in classroom discussion with one-word responses. Wyatt is beginning to build sentences using the carrier phrases (e.g., "I see the ____." "I like the ____."). During music activities, Wyatt is able to press preprogrammed icons to sing phrases of a song in response to a gestural prompt to use his iPad.

AAC Experience

Wyatt has been exposed to a myriad of AAC systems and interventions over the years. Beginning at a young age, he was introduced to picture exchange communication system (PECS), at which time intervention focused on developing communicative intent. Beginning in first grade, he was introduced to Language Acquisition through Motor Planning (LAMP) using a high-tech communication system funded through the school district. The LAMP, a therapeutic approach for children who are nonverbal or who have limited verbal abilities, utilizes principles of motor learning and the Unity® language program to teach children to communicate across environments. His success with this communication system was intermittent. He has been using his current AAC system for approximately the last six months.

Intervention

The primary purpose of Wyatt's participation in the intensive two-week intervention was to focus on expanding the purposes for which he communicates, increase his rate of responsiveness and initiations, and increase the mean number of symbols per message.

Description of Communication System

Wyatt's communication system consisted of an iPad2 with the Speak for Yourself app. Table 7–10 provides an overview of the skills that were specifically targeted during the two-week intense intervention program.

Response to Intervention

Wyatt made significant progress across the six days he attended camp. He demonstrated the ability to expand his greetings to other people, request a break during an activity, and comment during structured activities. He quickly learned new language constructions within various camp-themed activities following initial models. Upon the conclusion of camp, Wyatt was using two to three novel symbol messages to participate in group activities. Wyatt demonstrated eye contact when approaching peers and other adults in the room to greet or share his craft. Wyatt progressively demonstrated the ability to independently request squeezes to both his hands and head as a calming strategy. Providing sensory input assisted Wyatt in remaining on task and engaging in the various activities. Throughout camp, Wyatt acquired new vocabulary and created novel sentence constructions. Table 7–11 provides a summary of the words and phrases Wyatt mastered over the course of the two-week intervention program.

Suggestions and Recommendations

It is recommended that Wyatt continue to expand his greetings and comments to other settings with different peers and adults. It is further recommended that Wyatt continue to utilize his device to request a break in order to give him the opportunity to appropriately escape from a nonpreferred activity for a few minutes. This proactive strategy will allow Wyatt an opportunity to engage self-regulatory activities before returning to the activity. Because Wyatt learns new skills quickly, it is recommended that he be provided with the opportunities to generalize new skills across new settings with others early on in order to further expand his communication skills. The following strategies are suggested to facilitate Wyatt's ongoing acquisition of new skills:

◆ Model novel sentence constructions within the context of naturalistic interactions.
◆ Expand on Wyatt's communication attempts modeling for him more complex language forms.

Table 7–10. Summary of Wyatt's Response to the Intervention

PLOPs	Intervention Targets	Progress
Wyatt will carry his communication system when requested or prompted to do so by his one-on-one instructional aide.	Wyatt will independently transition his communication system throughout his day (*Operational*).	Wyatt's communication guide used a fading prompting approach to shift Wyatt away from being prompted dependent on this skill. Upon conclusion of the intervention program, Wyatt was independently transitioning his communication system in 80% of opportunities, and in the remaining opportunities, he was beginning to recognize the need to retrieve his communication system from the previous activity or environment.
Wyatt uses his communication system to answer simple yes/no questions and to request (e.g., I want chips) preferred food items, objects, and activities. Verbally, he responds with one-word utterances.	Wyatt will construct a minimum of three different 2- to 3-symbol language constructions (e.g., actor-action-object, action-object-location, negation, questions) to participate in group activities (*Linguistic*).	Upon completion of the two-week intensive intervention program, Wyatt was consistently using novel sentence constructions to participate in group activities (e.g., What that? Put it here, No more here). On the final day of camp, his mean number of symbols per message (MNSM) using his communication system was 2.7.
Wyatt currently works for preselected reinforcements requesting these items upon completion of a task using his communication system. Wyatt communicates the need to escape a stressful or nonpreferred activity using physical aggression (e.g., biting).	Wyatt will demonstrate the ability to utilize his communication system to initiate a request for a break during structured classroom activities, given a gestural cue from the clinician or support staff (*Strategic*).	Wyatt demonstrated progress towards this goal. Given a gestural cue, Wyatt initiated requests for a break during structured classroom activities in 8 out of 10 opportunities. During the last days of the two-week intervention, Wyatt was independently initiating a request for a break no less than two times over the course of each day.

Table 7–10. *continued*

PLOPs	Intervention Targets	Progress
When presented with an item he does not want, Wyatt will express "different" on his communication system to indicate he wants a different item or he does not like the presented item. Wyatt currently has difficulty initiating a comment on an activity. He requires multiple verbal prompts and models to select icons that will allow him to indicate a preference.	Wyatt will demonstrate the ability to utilize his communication system to comment on an activity (e.g., I like that, I don't like that, That was fun) with no more than 1 to 2 verbal prompts from the clinician or support staff in 8 out of 10 opportunities (*Social*).	Wyatt demonstrated significant progress in his ability to comment on an activity. When provided with a model, "I like that" and asked the question, "Do you like that?" Wyatt independently utilized his communication system to comment "I like that" on 3 out of 4 opportunities. Wyatt demonstrated the ability to comment, "I don't like that" when provided with a gestural cue on 3 out of 4 opportunities. Wyatt also demonstrated significant progress in his ability to comment, "I have that" independently in 5 out of 8 opportunities.
Wyatt will initiate a communicative interaction by tapping a person on the shoulder to gain their attention. He will occasionally respond to a wave within a structured setting. He is emerging in his ability to initiate an interaction with his instructional aide referencing them by name. Given multiple verbal prompts and models, he is beginning to initiate interactions with familiar peers.	Within 3 minutes of entering a new environment/activity and given no more than one gestural prompt, Wyatt will utilize his communication system to initiate a greeting or respond to a greeting posed by a peer, referencing them by name (e.g., "Hi Amanda") in 4 out of 5 opportunities (*Social*).	Wyatt used his communication system to initiate greetings with familiar adults and respond to greetings posed by peers in 60% of opportunities. In 40% of the opportunities, Wyatt benefitted from a partial prompt (i.e., guiding his hand with a touch of the elbow) or full prompt (i.e., hand-over-hand).

Table 7–11. Wyatt's Sentence Constructions and Vocabulary Acquired over the Course of the Two-Week Intervention Program

Sentence Constructions	New Core Vocabulary	New Fringe Vocabulary Sets
I see	On	Craft Vocabulary (e.g., paint)
I like	In	
I don't like	Up	Animals (e.g., dog, bunny)
Not that	It	
I make it	That	Astronomy words (e.g., earth, moon, star)
You make it	What	
I have that/it	Push	
Put on/in	Turn	
What	Little	
	Big	
	Pull	
	This	
	Help	
	Find	
	Good	
	Work	

- ◆ Scaffold communication opportunities throughout his day.
- ◆ Employ a faded prompting system to facilitate Wyatt's independent demonstration of new skills.

CONCLUSION

The case examples presented here illustrate the implementation of the intervention model that is the focus this book with a wide range of students, each with their unique intervention needs and AAC systems. They provide examples of different ways to write similar types of information. For example, how to describe a student's current means of communication or PLOPs in a positive manner. Too often, particularly in difficult cases, a student's abilities are presented by describing what they cannot do. The strategies and suggestions provided in this chapter can be adapted or modified based on the needs of your students. The case studies represented in this chapter illustrate the implementation of the intervention process from the initial intake of information through implementation with a group of students with CCNs who present with diverse intervention needs.

REFERENCE

Individuals with Disabilities Education Act, 20 U.S.C. § 1400. (2004).

APPENDIX A

Topics for Communication Guide Training

Training(s) for communication guides are customized based on their educational and professional background and the roles and responsibilities assigned to them. The following is a list of training topics to consider as you are developing your training including relevant chapters.

TRAINING TOPICS

Module 1: AAC Myths (Chapter 1)

Module 2: Communicative Competence (Chapter 1)

Module 3: Intervention as a Process (Chapter 2)

Module 4: Assessment—From Theory to Practice (Chapter 3)

Module 5: Importance of Vocabulary Selection (Chapter 4)

Module 6: Technical Aspects of Programming (Chapter 4)

Module 7: Programming to Support Acquisition of Communication (Chapter 4)

Module 8: Providing an Intensive Intervention (Chapter 5)

Module 9: Creating an Immersive Environment (Chapters 4 & 5)

Module 10: Proving a Socially Based Intervention by Creating Communication Opportunities (Chapters 4 & 5)

Module 11: Goal Development (Chapter 6)

Module 12: Progress Monitoring Strategies (Chapter 6)

APPENDIX B

Common Core Vocabulary

Core vocabulary refers to words used frequently in a variety of contexts, environments, and activities (Beukelman & Mirenda, 2014). These non-activity, non-environment-specific words have universal appeal because they are not context-specific. These words can be used across environments and activities. The majority of words we use to communicate on a daily basis are composed of core vocabulary (Banajee, Dicarlo, & Stricklin, 2003). Many core words have multiple meanings and can function as both nouns and verbs and even other forms of language including, adjectives, adverbs, determiners, and prepositions. The manner or context in which these words are used is helpful in recognizing what form of language they represent. For example, the message, "You get it" can be used to direct another person's behavior to physically grab or catch something. In this example, the word "you" is used in reference to who the communicator is talking to. But, these identical words can be used to also to indicate you understand something, "You get it!" In this example, the word "you" is being used in a more general reference. These subtle changes in use are important in demonstrating how students with CCNs are learning how to use their communication system for an expanding range of forms and functions. Recognizing the different ways in which a student uses a particular word is critical in documenting their progress. Table B–1 provides a list of some of the most commonly used core vocabulary words, and how novice AAC users apply these simple words to convey a variety of messages.

Table B–1. Core Vocabulary for Emergent Communicators

Core Word	Definition	Sample Use
Turn	*Verb:* to move in a circular motion (synonyms: spin, circle, rotate).	"Turn me" "Turn page"
	Verb: to change with respect to form or color, or to become something different.	"Turn blue" "Turn into a butterfly"
	Noun: the act of moving in a circular direction	"Take a turn"
	Noun: an opportunity to do something; usually successively after another person	"My turn"
Like	*Preposition:* having similar or identical characteristics; being alike	'Like me" "Walk like bear"
	Conjunction: in the same way	"Do it like you want it"
	Conjunction: as though; as if	"I don't feel like it"
	Noun: A person or object that is similar to another	"Like a dog"
	Adjective: sharing similar qualities to another person or thing	"Look like me"
	Verb: to indicate a preference for something; to indicate affirmation	"I like it" "No like popcorn"
Go	*Verb:* to travel or move from place to another	"I go there" "I go to class" "I go lunch"
	Verb: to depart or leave	"Go away"
	Noun: an attempt to do something	"Give it a go" "I go"
	Adjective: used to indicate something is functioning properly	"It go" "It no go"
Help	*Verb:* to assist someone	"I help" "You help" "No help"
	Noun: the action of assisting someone	"I want help" "Need help"
	Exclamation: to express urgency	"Help!"
Stop	*Verb:* to cease an action or event; to come to an end	""Stop it" "You stop" "No stop"
	Noun: to come to a standstill; end, finish	"Make it stop"

Table B–1. *continued*

Core Word	Definition	Sample Use
Eat	*Verb:* to consume or ingest	"Eat Cheerios"
	Noun: referring to foods or snacks	"What you eat" "Good eat"
Drink	*Verb:* to consume a liquid	"Drink juice"
	Noun: beverage	"I want drink" "Open drink" "No more drink"
You	*Pronoun:* used in reference to who the communicator is talking to	"You here?" "You do it"
	Pronoun: used as a general reference to any person	"You know it" "You get it"
I	*Pronoun:* used when referring to self	"I do it" "I want it"
That	*Pronoun:* used to by the speaker to reference someone or something observed or previously observed	"What that?" "That it" "I want that"
	Determiner: used before a noun to identify someone or something	"That car" "Not that book" "That him"
Want	*Verb:* used to request or to express desire for	"I want bubbles" "No want it"
	Noun: a long or craving for something	"What do you want" "I have want(s)"
What	*Pronoun:* used to request information	"What it?" "What do you want?
	Determiner: used before a noun to request information about a specific item or object	"What car?"
More	*Determiner:* used before a noun to indicate an additional amount	"Want more juice."
	Adverb: used as a comparative to indicate better than or the a greater extent	"More big"
My	*Determiner:* used before a noun to indicate possession	"My turn" "My truck"
	Determiner: used to express a sense of surprise or disbelief	"Oh my!"

continues

Table B–1. *continued*

Core Word	Definition	Sample Use
Here	*Adverb:* used to indicate a place or position	"Put here" "Go here" "Sit here"
	Adverb: used to introduce or draw attention to	"Look here" "Here it is"
	Exclamation: used to indicate presence	"I here"
	Exclamation: used to gain, attract, or direct someone's attention	"Here you take it" "Here I do it"
Again	*Adverb:* used to indicate recurrence	"Do it again" "Read again"
Do	*Verb:* to perform or execute	"I do it" "Do it again"
	Verb: to conduct oneself in a particular way	"Do like you want"
	Verb: used in questions and negative often before verbs	"What do you want?" "Do you like it?" "Do you have it?' "Do not like it"
It	*Pronoun:* a nondescript word used to refer to something	"Where is it?" "I like it"
All done	*Adjective:* used to indicate completion of a task or activity	"All done"
No/Not	*Determiner:* used to indicate the opposite, frequently in protest	"No want" "No like" "Not blue"
	Exclamation: used to indicate a negative response, frequently in response to a yes/no question	"No"
	Adverb: used to indicate not at all	"No more go"

REFERENCES

Banajee, M., Dicarlo, C., & Stricklin, S. B. (2003). Core vocabulary determination for toddlers. *Augmentative and Alternative Communication, 19,* 67–73.

Beukelman, D. R., & Mirenda, P. (2013). *Augmentative and alternative communication: Supporting children and adults with complex communication needs* (4th ed.). Baltimore, MD: Paul H. Brookes.

APPENDIX C

Books with
Repetitive Phrases

Table C–1 provides a list of popular children's stories with repetitive phrases and examples of how those repetitive phrases can be adapted using core vocabulary.

Table C–1. Books with Repetitive Phrases

Book Title	Author	Linguistic Targets	Repetitive Phrase	Modification to Target Core Vocabulary
Gallop!	Rufus Butler Seder	Like-Comparison	Can you gallop like a horse?	Can you gallop like a horse? I can!
Where's Spot?	Eric Hill	Question-Response Negation	Where's Spot. Not here.	Where is Spot? Not here!
Brown Bear, Brown Bear, What Do You See?	Eric Carle	Question-Response Commenting	What do you see? I see purple cat looking at me.	What do you see? I see purple cat looking at me.
Who Stole the Cookie from the Cookie Jar?	Various Authors	Question-Response Negation	Who stole the cookie from the cookie jar? Not me? Then Who?	Who took the cookie? Not me? Who?
Goodnight Moon	Margaret Wise Brown	Greetings	Good night kittens.	Go to sleep kittens.
The Very Hungry Caterpillar	Eric Carle	Feel	He was still hungry.	He feel hungry. He wanted more food.
From Head to Toe	Eric Carle	Question-Response Response	Can you do it?	I can do it!
Where Is My Frog?	Mercer Mayer	Question-Response	Where is my frog? No frog!	Where is my frog? Look in (log, grass, tree) Not here

Book Title	Author	Linguistic Targets	Repetitive Phrase	Modification to Target Core Vocabulary
I Want My Hat	Jon Klassen	Question-Response	I want my hat back.	I want my hat back!
		Possession	Have you seen my hat?	You see my hat?
				No hat here.
Go Away, Big Green Monster!	Ed Emberley	Attributes	Go away.	Go Away
				No Come back
Waiting Is Not Easy	Mo Williams	Question-Response	What is it?	What it?
			I cannot wait	I no (want) wait
			You will have to	You have to
				No more wait
If You Give a Mouse a Cookie	Laura Numeroff	Requesting	So he'll probably ask for . . .	He will ask for . . .
				He will want . . .
No, David	David Shannon	Negation	No, David	No do that

Seder, R. B. (2007). *Gallop: A scanimation picture book*. New York, NY: Workman Publishing Company; Hill, E. (2000). *Where's spot?* London, UK: Frederick Warne Publishers Ltd; Martin, B., & Carle, E. (1996). *Brown bear, brown bear what do you see?* New York, NY: Henry Holt and Co.; Brown, W. M. (2007). *Goodnight moon*. New York, NY: HarperCollins Publishers; Carle, E. (1981). *The very hungry caterpillar*. New York, NY: Philomel Books; Carle, E. (1999). *From head to toe*. New York, NY: HarperCollins Publishers; Mayer, M. (2010). *Where is my frog?* New York, NY: Sterling Publishing; Klassen, J. (2011). *I want my hat*. Somerville, MA: Candlewick Press; Emberley, E. (1992). *Go away, big green monster!* New York, NY: Little, Brown and Company; Williams, M. (2014). *Waiting is not easy*. New York, NY: Disney-Hyperion; Numeroff, L. (2002). *If you give a mouse a cookie*. New York, NY: HarperCollins Publishers; Shannon, D. (1998). *No, David*. Houston, TX: Blue Sky Press.

APPENDIX D

Adapted Stories: Creating Manageable Stories for Students with CCNs

Adapted stories are stories that have been modified in a manner that makes them physically, linguistically, and cognitively manageable for students with CCNs. Chapter 4, *Intervention Planning*, introduces the concept of adapting stories for students with CCNs; Chapter 5, *Intervention Implementation*, discusses how to implement shared reading experiences using these adapted stories. This appendix will provide specific examples of how three popular children's stories can be adapted to meet the needs of students who are learning to communicate with the support of AAC.

FROM HEAD TO TOE BY ERIC CARLE

Story Description

Students will be fully engaged in this interactive story by the popular children's author, Eric Carle. This story, which is presented in a predictable manner using repetitive statements, asks students if they can duplicate various movements demonstrated by different animals. Utilizing a question-response format, students are exposed to fringe words related to animals, actions, and body parts. The repetitive structure of this story gives students multiple exposure opportunities to core vocabulary words that are combined for the purposes of asking and responding to questions, directing the behavior of another person, and following simple directions.

Vocabulary

The following is a list of vocabulary words targeted throughout the story, and their frequency of occurrence. Core vocabulary words are noted with an asterisk.

Head to Toe Vocabulary

Pronouns	Actions	Objects	Possessions	Prepositions
I (37)*	can (25)*	head (1)	my (11)*	up (1)*
it (25)*	do (25)*	neck (1)		
you (12)*	turn (1)*	shoulders (1)		
	bend (1)	arms (1)		
	lift (1)	hands (1)		
	clap (1)	chest (1)		
	hit (1)	back (1)		
	arch (1)	hips (1)		
	wiggle (2)	knees (1)		
	bend (1)	legs (1)		
	kick (1)	feet (1)		
	stomp (1)	toe (1)		

Story Adaptations

This book can be bought in a board form, which is highly recommended. Suggested page fluffers include foam cutouts, Popsicle sticks, and/or colorful paper clips. The greeting "hi" can be added to the story language to give students practice initiating and responding to greetings. The sentence, "I raise my shoulders" was changed to, "I lift my shoulders up." Another option would be to replace "I can do it" with "my turn" if your goal is to target this message construction. The story text is easily adapted. The original text can be used with little modification other than adding picture symbols. The following phrases are repeated throughout the story:

I am a (insert animal name)

I (action word) my (insert body part)

Can you do it?

I can do it.

Reading Strategies

Prior to Reading the Story

1. Introduce zoo animals using manipulatives and have students brainstorm vocabulary related to visiting the zoo. Have students bring in photographs or pictures of various zoo animals and compare real-life zoo animals to picture symbols represented in the book.
2. Give students an opportunity to practice labeling body parts on themselves and their favorite stuffed animal. Have students touch or point to specific body parts when shown specific picture symbols (e.g., point to neck). You can also focus your instruction on the word "my" by giving students directives such as "touch my nose." Then you can flip it around and have students respond to questions using "my" by asking them, "Whose foot is this?"

While Reading the Text

1. Program single message devices such as a BIGMack with "Can you do it," and another with "I can do it" in order to facilitate answering and responding to questions.
2. Identify familiar and unfamiliar core vocabulary. Practice using repetitive phrases (e.g., "my turn") while reading the book by having students request turns to turn pages or model the actions of the animals.
3. Give students practice imitating action words, pairing verbal directions with picture symbols. Gently motor students through actions to let them experience the action themselves.

After Reading the Text

1. Ask students simple comprehension questions and offer answer choices with the use of picture symbols. Describe the characteristics of the zoo animals and/or children present in the story.
2. Game: *Who does it?* Present students with the question "Who ____ their ____?" and fill in an action and body part. Provide students with three visuals of different animals that they can select to answer.
3. Reinforce action words by picking one to two action words each day to target. Students will use these actions to manipulate a variety of objects. For example, one day students can turn things such as tops, lids on bottles, sit-n-spin, pinwheels, while on another day they can bend things such as straws, pool noodles, and red vines.
4. Music: Have students sing and move to *Head, Shoulders, Knees, and Toes*. Don't forget to provide visuals for each movement. Ask students to identify their own body parts as an introduction to the song (e.g., "Show me your head," or "Point to your head").

5. Song: *There's a Spider on the Floor* ("There's a spider on my arm, on my arm"). Have students sing this song with the use of visuals to incorporate different body parts and locations where a spider can be.

SNOWY DAY BY EZRA JACK KEATS

Story Description

This Caldecott Medal award-winning story follows a boy named Peter and his adventures through a snowy day in the city. Peter participates in a snowball fight, shakes snow off a tree, and pretends to be a mountain climber. This is a great book to use to introduce winter vocabulary, different types of weather, and to discover the power of a little boy's imagination. This story models the use of core vocabulary for the main communicative purposes of commenting and expressing simple emotions using a variety of sentence patterns including subject + verb and subject + verb + object.

Vocabulary

The following is a list of vocabulary words targeted throughout the story and their frequency of occurrence. Core vocabulary words are noted with an asterisk.

Snowy Day Vocabulary

Pronouns	Actions	Prepositions	Objects	Emotions	Auxiliary Words
I (1)*	go (10)*	down (2)	snow (10)	happy (1)	more (7)*
	make (2)*	up (2)	snowball (1)	sad (1)	there (1)*
	play (6)*	on (1)*	snowman (1)		all done (3)*
	stop (1)*	in (4)*	head (1)		again (1)*
	see (1)*		water (1)		not (1)*
					more (1)*

Story Adaptations

This story was adapted to meets the needs of emergent communicators to help give them a sense of story. The original story, although delightful, will be overwhelming for students with cognitive impairments and significant delays in receptive language. It is just too much language! Therefore, the story text was significantly modified while preserving the story content and themes. Refer to Table D–1 for suggestions on how to modify the story text. Suggested page fluffers include small- or medium-sized puff balls that are glued to pages to create a space between them, making it easier for those who find manipulating pages challenging.

Reading Strategies

Prior to Reading the Story

1. Have students sort winter and summer clothes into baskets.
2. Have students take turns trying on winter clothes.
3. Have students bring in photos of themselves playing in the snow.

While Reading the Text

1. Students can use their communication system to match the symbols presented throughout the story.
2. A single message output device can be pre-programmed to say, "go" and student can push it each time Peter goes walking in the story and when the student sees the picture icon for "go" or "more go."

After Reading the Text

1. Use follow-up activities to reinforce new vocabulary: To reinforce the new vocabulary of "snow," "snowman," "snowball," "water," "head," "see," and "all gone," a picture bingo game can be used. Printed picture icons for each vocabulary word can be glued onto a blank bingo card worksheet. The facilitating adult calls out icons one by one. Students find the vocabulary on their bingo card and mark it with a bingo chip or highlighter. If applicable, students can also find the called-out word on their communication device.
2. Use follow-up activities to reinforce specific sentence patterns: To reinforce the sentence pattern of "more go" and "stop," students can play freeze dance with music. Music is played and communication guide models, "more go" while holding corresponding picture icons for "more" and "go" or directing students' attention to these words on their own devices. Students dance or shake musical instruments (e.g., tambourine or maracas) while music is being played. When the communication guide stops the music and says, "stop," simultaneously holding a picture icon for "stop," students will freeze and hold their position until the

Table D–1. Adapted Story Text: *Snowy Day* by Ezra Jack Keats

Page(s)	Original Story Text	Adapted Text
Pages 1–2	One winter morning . . . (picture of little boy looking out window)	I see snow.
Pages 3–4	After breakfast . . . (picture of little boy walking out side looking at a mound of snow)	More snow. I like snow.
Page 5	Crunch, crunch, crunch, . . . (picture of footprints in snow)	Go, go, go
Page 6	He walked with . . . (picture of little boy looking back at the footprints he just made in the snow)	Look! I made footprints.
Pages 7–8	Then he dragged . . . (picture of snow with lines in snow from little boy dragging his feet in the snow)	Go, go, go
Pages 9–10	It was a stick.. (pictures of boy with a stick trying to knock the snow down out of the tree)	Snow up. Snow come down.
Page 11	Down fell the . . . (picture of boy with snow on his head)	Snow down.
Page 12	(picture of boy walking away)	Time to go play.
Pages 13–14	He thought it . . . (picture of boys having a snowball fight)	I don't like.
Page 15	So he made . . . (picture of snowman)	I made a happy snowman.
Page 16	And he made . . . (picture of boy making snow angels in the snow)	I like.
Page 17	He pretended he . . . (picture of little boy climbing up mound of snow).	Go up.
Page 18	And he slid . . . (picture of little boy sliding down the mound of snow)	Go down.
Page 19	He picked up . . . (picture of little boy holding a ball of snow)	I take snow.
Page 20	He told his . . . (picture of little boy talking to his mother)	Play all done.

Table D–1. *continued*

Page(s)	Original Story Text	Adapted Text
Pages 21–22	And he thought . . . (picture of little boy taking a bath)	Time to take bath.
Page 23	Before he got . . . (picture of little boy reaching in the pocket of his jacket looking for the snowball he had put in there)	Uh oh! Snow all gone.
Page 24	(picture of boy sleeping)	Sleep.
Page 25	While he slept, . . . (picture of sun)	Snow all gone.
Page 26	But when he . . . (picture of boy waking up)	I see snow I like snow
Pages 27–28	After breakfast he . . . (picture of little boy and his friend standing outside in the snow)	More play
Back Cover		All done

Source: 1976, New York, NY: Puffin Books.

music is turned back on and communication guide says and models "more go."

3. Use follow-up activities to reinforce communication purposes modeled throughout the story: To reinforce the communication purpose of commenting on other people's actions, the students will look at the various children's books and comment on what each character is doing in the story. For example, the child can look at the book *If You Give a Mouse a Cookie* and comment on what the mouse is doing (e.g., "more go," "eat," "stop"). This can be repeated with any other children's story.

4. Make snow using a shaved ice machine and let students make their own snowballs. Encourage students to bring in gloves or mittens from home.

GALLOP! BY RUFUS BUTLER SEDER

Story Description

In this Scanimation picture book, Rufus Butler Seder relates the story of how animals move. On each page, the reader can actually watch the animals move, as the illustrations are animated. He asks the reader if they can move like a certain animal. This story teaches the students how to use the word "like" for the purpose of comparing two things. This story further models the use of core vocabulary for different communicative purposes, including asking questions and making statements using a variety of different sentence patterns (e.g. subject + verb, subject+ predicate+ object, and questioning).

Vocabulary

The following is a list of vocabulary words targeted throughout the story and their frequency of occurrence. Core vocabulary words are noted with an asterisk.

Gallop Vocabulary

Pronouns	Verbs	Nouns	Auxiliary Words
I (8)*	can (17)*	horse (1)	are (2)
you (10)*	like (8)*	rooster (1)	is (1)
it(1)*	do (1)*	dog (1)	what (1)*
	gallop (2)	cat (1)	and (1)
	walk (2)	chimp (1)	that (1)*
	jump (2)	butterfly (1)	all (1)*
	run(2)	eagle (1)	
	fly (3)	turtle (1)	
	swing (2)	star (1)	
	swim (2)		
	feel (1)*		

Story Adaptations

This book comes in board book format and it is strongly recommended that this version be used. Some of the actions that were used were adapted to use less abstract vocabulary. For example, the original story text states, "Can you *strut* like a rooster?" "Strut" was changed to "walk." Also "flutter" and "soar" were changed to "fly." Overall, the conceptual format was not altered. Table D–2 provides suggestions on how to modify the story text. Suggested page fluffers include binder clips or foam stickers.

Table D–2. Adapted Story Text: *Gallop: A Scanimation Picture Book* by Rufus Butler Seder

Page(s)	Original Story Text	Adapted Text
Pages 1–2	Can you gallop like a horse? Giddy up-a-loo	Can you gallop like a horse? I can!
Page 18	If you can soar . . .	You can fly. You can swim. You can swing.
Page 19	Then take a bow . . .	You can do it all! Feel proud like a star!

Source: 2007, New York, NY: Workman Publishing Company.

Reading Strategies

Prior to Reading the Story

1. Introduce students to the animals that will be referred to in the story. Show the students objects or pictures of these animals.
2. Introduce students to different actions. Use a game such as "Simon Says," and ask students to act out or imitate different movements (e.g., gallop, fly, jump, swim), pairing verbal directives with picture symbols.
3. Have students match the action with the picture of the animal.

While Reading the Text

1. Have students request turns to turn pages as you read the book.
2. Have students answer simple comprehension questions using their AAC device such as, "What animal can gallop?" Answer: "horse"; or "Can you run?" Answer: "I can!"
3. Pass out animals that will appear in the story so students can participate in telling the story. When their animal appears in the story, they can stand up and say (using their AAC system), "I have it!" or "That my animal!"

After Reading the Text

1. Present students with objects of the animals in the story in a field of three. Give the direction, "horse," or "Show me turtle," and students will point to the object.

2. Ask students to manipulate the objects to match what they do in the story. Give the direction, "Make horse run" or "Show me cat jump."
3. Ask students to perform the action themselves. Give the directive (paired with symbols of course), "Fly like butterfly," "Swing like Chimp."
4. Ask the students, "Can you jump like a cat?" and have students use their AAC device to say, "I can."

BROWN BEAR, BROWN BEAR BY ERIC CARLE

Story Description

This children's classic is a fictional story about different animals and what they see through the use of repetitive phrases "What do you see?" and "I see a ____." In this picture book, Eric Carle helps the reader associate colors and meanings to objects using repetitive phrases and colorful pictures of animals. This story teaches emergent AAC communicators how to use the word "see" to describe objects and colors. This story further models the use of core vocabulary (i.e., you, I, do, and what) for different communicative purposes, including asking questions and making statements using a variety of different sentence patterns (e.g., subject + verb, subject+ predicate+ object, and questioning.

Vocabulary

The following is a list of vocabulary targeted throughout the story and their frequency of occurrence. Core vocabulary words are noted with an asterisk.

Brown Bear, Brown Bear Vocabulary

Pronouns	Actions	Animals	People	Colors	Auxiliary Words
you (10)*	do (11)*	bear (2)	children (2)	brown (3)	what (11)*
I (9)*	see (22)*	bird (3)	teacher (3)	red (3)	
		duck (3)		yellow (3)	
		horse (3)		blue (3)	
		frog (3)		green (3)	
		car (3)		purple (3)	
		dog (3)		white (3)	
		sheep (3)		black (3)	
		fish (3)		gold (3)	

Story Adaptations

This book comes in many different formats including board books. The overall conceptual format was not altered. In the original format the repetitive phrase "I see (color + animal) precedes the picture of the animal referenced. This can be confusing for the student with CCNs because the story text does not match the illustrations. Moving this text to the page with the corresponding animal makes the story more linguistically and cognitively manageable for the student. Additionally, do not feel you have to repeat the symbols on the page. For example, instead of having symbols for each word (e.g., brown-bear-brown-bear) have these symbols represented one time (e.g., brown bear) and the reader can simply point to the symbols twice. Suggested page fluffer: To reduce the difficulty of turning pages, small clothespins can be cut in half and secured between the pages to separate them and make them easier to turn (Table D–3).

Reading Strategies

Prior to Reading the Story

1. Introduce students to the animals that are referred to in the story. Show students objects or pictures of the animals.
2. Introduce students to different colors. Have students receptively and/or expressively identify the colors presented.
3. Bring pictures of the animals and the colors. Have students match the color with the animal.

While Reading the Text

1. Have students take turns turning the pages while using their AAC system to indicate "my turn," "your turn." This will reinforce turn-taking.

Table D–3. Adapted Story Text: *Brown Bear, Brown Bear What Do You See?* By Bill Martin Jr. and Eric Carle

Page(s)	Original Text	Adapted Story Text
Pages 1–2	Picture of Brown Bear	Brown Bear, What do you see?
Pages 2–3	Picture of Red Bird	I see red bird. Red bird, What do you see?

Source: 1996, New York, NY: Henry Holt and Co.

2. Have students answer simple comprehension questions using their AAC device such as "What does brown bear see?" Answer: "red bird," or "What color is the bird?" Answer: "red."
3. Give students animals corresponding with the animals in the story. They can participate in telling the story. Additionally, the communication guide can ask students, "Who has (color + animal)?" to which students can respond, "I have it!"

After Reading the Text

1. Present students with objects of the animals in the story in a field of three. Give the direction, "Find bear," or "Show me frog," and students will point to the object.
2. Ask students to color a picture of the different animals in the story. Give the direction, "Color the bear brown," or "Which crayon do you need to color the bird?"
3. Have students use their AAC device to answer yes/no questions. "Is the bear red?" or "Is the frog green?"

APPENDIX E

Sample Activities and Lessons

Students with CCNs respond best when activities and lessons are engaging, motivating, and relevant. The following are sample activities/lessons that have proven very successful when working with students with CCNs.

ACTIVITY/LESSON #1: BUBBLES

Overview of Activity

This is an activity that is enjoyed by students of all ages. Students are fully engaged making bubbles, using bubbles wands of different shapes and sizes. This activity encourages students to use their communication system to direct the behavior of their peers and familiar adults (e.g., "You pop," "You get it"), request help, request objects, and comment about the activity (e.g., "I made bubbles," "I like bubbles"). While they are busy creating and popping bubbles, students use core vocabulary to construct messages 1 to 3 words in length.

Materials

Bubble soap/solution and bubble wands (cookie cutters, strawberry baskets, plastic soda holder, hangers bent into shapes)

Facilitating Communicative Competence

Operational Competence Targets

This activity begins by having students transition from their current activity or task to the location where bubble activity will take place. This gives students an additional opportunity to transfer their communication system from one location to the next. Students who are using dynamic display-type systems will have multiple opportunities to navigate through their system to find activity-related folders (e.g., core page, activity page, color page), construct sentences, and activate the message bar. Students will access symbols using their preferred or targeted access method (e.g., direct select, scanning).

Linguistic Competence Targets

In addition to expanding their use and knowledge of core vocabulary, students will be introduced to activity-specific fringe words. They will learn how to use the words "blow" and "pop" as action words, and how to distinguish between bubbles using the attributes big and little. Access to core vocabulary and fringe words will give students the opportunity to formulate messages of increasing length and complexity.

Vocabulary. The following is a list of words typically elicited and modeled through this activity. Any modification or extension of this activity has the potential to expand this list. Core vocabulary words are noted with an asterisk.

Pronouns	Actions	Objects	Prepositions & Attributes	Auxiliary Words
I*	Open*	Basket	Sticky	More*
You*	Go*	Cookie cutter	Big*	All done*
It*	Stop*		Little*	No*
	Pop	Bubbles	In*	
	Blow	Wand		
	Look*			
	Want*			
	Open*			

Language Constructions. The following is a list of the language constructions typically elicited from students and modeled by communication guides throughout this activity.

Two-Symbol Language Constructions	Three-Symbol Language Constructions
Actor-Action	Actor-Action-Object
Action-Object	Action-Location-Object
Action-Location	Action-Adjective-Object
Negation	Action-Quantity-Object
Attribute-Object	Formulate question
Formulate question	

One, Two, and Three-Plus Symbol Messages

One Symbol	Two Symbols	Three or More Symbols
Go	Want bubbles?	Put wand in
Stop	Want pop?	I want bubbles
Want	Need open	You get bubbles
More	More bubbles	I get bubbles
Pop	Big bubble	I want more
Help	Little bubble	I want pop
All Done	Pop bubble	Help pop bubbles
Bubbles	Want open?	I need help
Open	Want close?	I want open
Close	You close	More pop bubbles
Blow	I open	Get more bubbles
Sticky	Get bubbles	I need wand
Big	Need wand	Want big bubbles
Little	Wand in	Pop more bubbles
More	See bubbles	Get little bubbles
Look	Pop it	I like bubbles
Basket	Like bubbles	Like pop it
Wand	Want bubbles	Bubbles are sticky
No	Want basket	I want basket
	Pop it	
No	It sticky	Help me pop
	All done	All done pop

One Symbol	Two Symbols	Three or More Symbols
	Stop pop	Stop pop bubbles
	Yes bubbles	No like bubbles
	Want more?	Do you like?
	Don't want	I want that
		Don't want that

Social Competence Targets

Students will have the opportunity to participate in a variety of communicative exchanges, both as responders and as initiators. Students will use their communication for a variety of communicative purposes throughout the activity including to request objects, direct the behavior of another person, cease the action of another person, request assistance, reject an object, express a preference, describe action of self (or other), and respond to requests for information.

Strategic Competence Targets

Throughout this activity, students will have opportunities to gain the attention of the adult leading the activity to request items necessary to complete the task and comment about the activity itself. The activity will naturally lend itself to providing students with opportunities to clarify messages that are purposefully misinterpreted. The adult leading the activity can also fail to respond to students' communicative attempts requiring them to practice persistency or modifying their message to ensure that it is received by the facilitating adults.

Activity Steps and Sample Language

This activity begins by explaining to students what it is they are going to be doing. At this time you may even want to model the activity. Communication guides may ask students various questions including, "What do we need?" "We need . . . " "Do we need?" Do you have it?" The communication guide may purposefully hold up an item irrelevant to the activity and ask students, "Do we need this?" giving students an opportunity to practice answering yes/no questions. One alteration to this activity would be to actually make the bubble solution with the students. This would add an additional layer of communication opportunities for the students.

Throughout the activity communication guides create communication opportunities using communication temptations (e.g., handing student container of bubbles they are unable to open), ask questions using aided language stimulation, and model language for participation including the use of requests and comments. The student can request to blow bubbles themselves or request their communication guide to blow bubbles for them. Students can even direct the behaviors of peers instructing them to blow or pop bubbles. An extension to this activity would be to set a timer and have students pop as many bubbles as they can before the timer stops. If you really want to create a sea of bubbles, use a floor fan and larger wand to inundate students with bubbles. This can be really fun and really gets the students excited about this activity.

ACTIVITY/LESSON #2: SCOOTER BOARDS

Overview of Activity

This is a simple activity students really enjoy. In its simplest form students sit on their scooter boards and direct an adult (or peer) to pull them around a room. A variation of the activity has students transport a beanbag from a Hula-Hoop at one end of the play space to the other end while being pulled by a familiar adult or peer. Students can also instruct the familiar adult or peer to direct them through an obstacle course. This activity has endless possibilities. This activity encourages students to use their communication to direct the behavior of another person, request help, request continuation of a preferred activity, make object requests, and comment about the activity. This activity will reinforce their use of core vocabulary through their ability to communicate using various 1 to 3-word phrases that include both core and fringe vocabulary.

Materials

Scooter boards, rope, optional items (e.g., beanbags—different colors, Hula-Hoops, cones, ramp)

Facilitating Communicative Competence

Operational Competence Targets

The activity will begin by making sure students have their communication systems available. Students with dynamic display type systems will have multiple opportunities to navigate through their system to find activity-related folders (e.g., core page, activity page, color page), construct sentences, and activate the message bar. Students will be able to access symbols using their preferred or targeted access method (e.g., direct select, scanning). Communication systems, including high-tech communication systems and non-tech communication boards and book, can be situated on the scooter boards right in front of the student ready to be used. For students using low-tech communication boards, consider adhering communication boards directly on the scooter boards using self-laminating sheets.

Linguistic Competence Targets

In addition to expanding their use and knowledge of core vocabulary, students will be introduced to activity-specific fringe words. They will learn how to use the words "pull" and "push" as action words as well as using colors as attributes (e.g., green beanbag). Access to core vocabulary and fringe words will give students the opportunity to formulate messages of increasing length and complexity.

Vocabulary. The following is a list of words typically elicited and modeled through this activity. Any variations of this activity have the potential to expand this list. Core vocabulary words are marked with an asterisk.

Pronouns	Actions	Objects	Prepositions	Auxiliary Words
I*	Push	Scooter board	On*	No*
You*	Pull	Beanbag	Off*	More*
My*	Go*	Hula-Hoop	In*	Help*
It*	Stop*	Rope		
	Turn*			
	Want*			
	Get*			
	Put*			
	Do*			
	Like*			

Language Constructions. The following is a list of the language constructions typically elicited and modeled throughout this activity.

Two-Symbol Language Constructions	Three-Symbol Language Constructions
Actor-Action	Actor-Action-Object
Action-Object	Action-Location-Object
Action-Location	Action-Adjective-Object
Negation	Action-Quantity-Object
Attribute-Object	Formulate question
Formulate question	

One, Two, and Three-Plus Symbol Messages. The following is a sample of one, two, and three-plus symbol messages students may use and communications guides may model throughout this activity:

One Symbol	Two Symbols	Three or More Symbols
Go	Get more	I want push
No	Put in	My turn pull
Stop	More push	Get on scooter
Want	Go push	You push/pull scooter
More	Stop push	I push/pull scooter
Help	More pull	I get it
Get	I pull	Put in Hula-Hoop
Beanbag	Stop pull	Get more beanbag
Push	Want more?	More beanbag in
Rope	No more	You want more?
Turn	Get it	I do it
Beanbag	You help	You do it
Scooter	All done	You like it?
Hula-Hoop	Get on	Put in more beanbag
	Get off	Turn me more
	My turn	You help me
	Your turn	My turn scooter
	Get rope	You turn it
	Push scooter	I got (color) beanbag
	What color?	I all done
	(Color) beanbag	I like to push/pull
	Hold beanbag	Do you like it?
	Turn me	Push/pull me more
	You hold	Put in lap
		I hold it

Social Competence Targets

Students will have the opportunity to participate in a variety of communicative exchanges, both as responders and initiators. Students will use their communication for a variety of communicative purposes throughout the activity including requesting objects, directing the behavior of another person, ceasing the action of another person, requesting assistance, rejecting an object, expressing a preference, describing action of self (or other), and responding to requests for information.

Strategic Competence Targets

Throughout the activity, students will have opportunities to gain the attention of other students and familiar adults. This activity has the potential to give students multiple opportunities to clarify messages that are purposefully misinterpreted. Communication guides can create opportunities for students to practice persistence and to recognize when and how to modify their messages for clarification as communication guides intentionally fail to respond to the students' communicative attempts or misinterpret their requests.

Activity

Begin by introducing students to activity and related fringe vocabulary. Demonstrate the activity including how to use their AAC system to direct the person who will be pulling them across the room on their scooter board. Give students an opportunity to select which scooter board they want to ride on and identify who will be their puller (sample language: "Want on scooter," "Sit on scooter," "sit down," "You pull," "Hold rope," "Who's turn?," "Your turn," "My turn"). There may be a student who prefers to just watch and not necessarily partake in this activity and that is perfectly fine. Their communication guide will simply follow their lead. There will be multiple opportunities for the communication guide to employ various language stimulation techniques. Frequently, these are the students who in turn want to be the pullers or helpers. It is the communication guide's responsibility to get the student engaged in the activity through their own excitement of the activity.

Variation #1

One variation to this activity is to incorporate Hula-Hoops and beanbags. Set up Hula-Hoops on either side of the play space and place all of the beanbags inside Hula-Hoops on one side of the room. Place scooter boards on the other side of the room next to the Hula-Hoops without the beanbags. This will be the side students start from. The adult leading the activity says, "Ready, set . . . " and waits for student to initiate "go" before pulling the student across the room to get the first beanbag. Once at the other end of the room, student picks up the beanbag or instructs their communication guide or peer to get it and turn them around so they can head back to the original Hula-Hoop where they will put the beanbag. This sequence is repeated until all of the beanbags have been moved from one hula-hoop to the other. Throughout this activity communication guides elicit and model AAC use. Sample language: "more go," "no stop," "turn me," "scooter no go," "get beanbag," "my turn," "you turn," "turn it/scooter."

Variation #2

A second variation to this activity is to set up an obstacle course using cones, furniture, hula-hoops, and ramps. Consider creating a bridge for students to maneuver under. Students direct pullers in navigating them through the obstacle course.

ACTIVITY/LESSON #3: SENSORY BAGS

Overview of Activity

This is a great activity that students will not only enjoy making but playing with afterward. Students will make sensory fish bags by filling a plastic Ziploc bag with hair gel, glitter, and foam fish. This activity will encourage students to use their communication to direct the behavior of another person, request help, make object requests, and comment about the activity. This activity will reinforce their use of core vocabulary through their ability to communicate using various one- to three-word phrases that include both core and fringe vocabulary.

Materials

Ziploc bags, blue hair gel, scoop (big and little), foam fish (different sizes and colors), glitter (different colors), packing tape, and scissors

Facilitating Communicative Competence

Operational Competence Targets

The activity will begin by making sure the student has their communication system available and turned on, if applicable. Students with dynamic display-type systems will have multiple opportunities to navigate through their system to find activity-related folders (e.g., core page, activity page, color page), construct sentences, and activate the message bar. Students will have multiple opportunities to navigate through their AAC system. Students will be able to access symbols using their preferred or targeted access method (e.g., direct select, scanning).

Linguistic Competence Targets

In addition to expanding their use and knowledge of core vocabulary, students will be introduced to activity-specific fringe words. They will learn how to use the word "scoop" as both an action word and object label, the word "squish" as an action word and as an attribute, and how to distinguish between objects using the attributes big and little ("I want big scoop"). Access to core vocabulary and fringe words will give students the opportunity to formulate messages of increasing length and complexity.

Vocabulary. The following is a list of words typically elicited and modeled through this activity. Any modification or extension has the potential to expand this list. Core vocabulary words are noted with an asterisk.

Pronouns	Actions	Objects	Prepositions & Attributes	Auxiliary Words
I*	Stop	Bag	In*	No*
You*	Want*	Glitter	(colors)	More*
It*	Get*	Fish		Help*
	Open*	Gel		All done*
	Shake	Jar		Here*
	Close	Scoop		That*
	Squish	Tape		
	Scoop			
	Tape			
	Like*			
	Do*			
	Put*			

Language Constructions. The following is a list of the language constructions typically elicited from students and modeled by communication guides throughout this activity:

Two-Symbol Language Constructions	Three-Symbol Language Constructions
Actor-Action	Actor-Action-Object
Action-Object	Action-Location-Object
Action-Location	Action-Adjective-Object
Negation	Action-Quantity-Object
Attribute-Object	Formulate question
Formulate question	

One, Two, and Three or More-Symbol Messages. The following is a list of one, two, and three-plus symbol constructions that can be elicited from the AAC user or modeled by the communication guide.

One-Symbol Messages	Two-Symbol Messages	Three or More-Symbol Messages
No	Close bag	I want gel
Stop	Tape bag	I want glitter
Want	More gel	I want fish
More	More glitter	I want more
Help	More fish	Want help open?
Get	No more	I help you
Bag	Squish bag	I like it!
Open	You like?	I squish it!
Shake	Want more?	Want more gel
Glitter	No more	You want more?
Fish	Fish bag	I do it
Gel	You help	You do it
All Done	Get bag	You like it?
Jar	Open bag	Put in more
Close	Open jar	Get blue gel
Squish	Scoop gel	Put in here
Scoop	Close jar	You scoop gel
Tape	Get glitter	Scoop more gel
	Shake glitter	Shake more glitter
	No more	I all done glitter
	All done	I want that scoop
	More tape	Do you like it?

Social Competence Targets

Students will have the opportunity to participate in a variety of communicative exchanges, both as responders and initiators. Students will use their communication for a variety of communicative purposes throughout the activity including requesting objects, directing the behavior of another person, ceasing the action of another person, requesting assistance, rejecting an object, expressing a preference, describing action of self (or other), and responding to requests for information

Strategic Competence Targets

Throughout the activity students will have opportunities to gain the attention of the adult leading the activity to request items necessary to complete the task and comment about the activity itself. The activity will naturally lend itself to providing the student with opportunities to clarify messages that are purposefully misinterpreted. The adult leading the activity can also fail to respond to the students' communicative attempts, requiring them to practice persistency or modifying their message.

Activity

Step #1

Reinforce the zip-lock bag with tape. This step can be completed ahead of time or with the assistance of student(s).

Step #2

Scoop hair gel into bag. Sample language: "Open hair gel," "Want big scoop," "I want big scoop," "More scoop," "Not that scoop," "Want open gel," "Help me open," "Want gel," "I want gel," "More gel," "I like/don't like gel," "Stop," "No more," "all done gel"

Step #3

Add foam fish and glitter. Sample language: "Want (color) fish," "How many fish?," "(number) fish in bag," "get more fish," "get glitter," "I want glitter," "You/I shake glitter," "More glitter," "Stop shake," "Go," "shake, shake, shake."

Step #4

Help the child fold the bag while pushing the air out, then seal the bag with tape. Sample language: "Push bag," "Help me push," "You push," "Get tape," "Need more tape," "Little or big tape?," "Want little tape," "Sticky tape," "All done bag."

Step #5

Play! Have the child explore the feel of the bag as they push on it, feel the gel move, and see the fish and glitter swirl in the bag. Sample language: "Look fish," "I see glitter," "It squishy," "I like/don't like," "Make more," "All done bag."

ACTIVITY/LESSON #4: SLIME

Overview of Activity

This is a great activity that students will enjoy making and playing with afterward. Students will mix together a variety of ingredients to create slime. They will incorporate googly eyes and shapes as they play with slime to make different creatures. This activity will encourage students to use their communication to direct the behavior of another person, request help, make object requests, and comment about the activity. This activity will reinforce their use of core vocabulary through their ability to communicate using various one- to three-word phrases that include both core and fringe vocabulary.

Materials

Colored Elmer's Glitter Glue, 1 cup water, 1 tsp. Borax, 1 Tbsp. water, tub, googly eyes, cookie cutters

Facilitating Communicative Competence

Operational Competence Targets

This activity will begin by making sure the student has their communication system available and turned on if applicable. Students with dynamic display-type systems will have multiple opportunities to navigate through their system to find activity-related folders (e.g., core page, activity page, color page), construct sentences and activate the message bar. Students will have multiple opportunities to navigate through their AAC system. Students will be able to access symbols using their preferred or targeted access method (e.g., direct select, scanning).

Linguistic Competence Targets

In addition to expanding their use and knowledge of core vocabulary, students will be introduced to activity-specific fringe words. They will learn how to use the word "squish" as both an action word and attribute label to describe the slime. Access to core vocabulary and fringe words will give students the opportunity to formulate messages of increasing length and complexity.

Vocabulary. The following is a list of words typically elicited and modeled through this activity with additional words listed in the examples of one, two, and three or more-symbol messages. Any modification or extension of this activity has the potential to expand this list. Core vocabulary words are noted with an asterisk.

Pronouns	Actions	Objects	Prepositions	Auxiliary Words
I*	Pour	Water	In*	More*
You*	Get*	Slime	On*	Help*
It*	Look	Bottle		Here*
	Feel*	Glue		No*
	Squish	Eyes		
	Like*	Glitter		
	Glue	Cup		
	See	Borax/powder		
	Want*			
	Need*			
	Look			
	Do*			
	Open*			
	Close			
	Turn*			

Language Constructions, The following is a list of the language constructions typically elicited from students and modeled by communication guides throughout this activity.

Two-Symbol Language Constructions	Three-Symbol Language Constructions
Actor-Action	Actor-Action-Object
Action-Object	Action-Location-Object
Action-Location	Action-Adjective-Object
Negation	Action-Quantity-Object
Attribute-Object	Formulate question
Formulate question	

One, Two, and Three-Symbol Messages. The following is a sample of one, two, and three-plus symbol messages students may use and communications guides may model throughout this activity:

One-Symbol Messages	Two-Symbol Messages	Three Or More-Symbol Messages
Open	More water	I see glitter
Close	More glue	Pour water in
Yes	Pour in	Pour in cup
No	I see	Put it here
Stop	Stop pour	I feel slime
In	Water in	I need help
Help	Help me	No more glue
Pour	Get water	Water in tub
Water	More slime	I want more
Get	Look here	Pour Borax/powder in
Look	I do	I like slime
Feel	Squish it	I no like
Slime	Eyes on	No like slime
Squish	Feel slime	I do it
More	Put on	Put eyes on it
Like	Need bottle	I make shape
Bottle	Squish slime	I see slime
Glue		You squish it
		I squish it

Social Competence Targets

Students will have the opportunity to participate in a variety of communicative exchanges both as a respondent and initiator. Students will use their communication for a variety of communicative purposes throughout the activity including requesting objects, directing the behavior of another person, ceasing the action of another person, requesting assistance, requesting an object, expressing a preference, describing an action of self (or other), responding to requests for information

Strategic Competence Targets:

In this activity students will have opportunities to gain the attention of the adult leading the activity to request items necessary to complete the task and comment about the activity itself. The activity will naturally lend itself to providing the student with opportunities to clarify messages that are purposefully misinterpreted. The adult leading the activity can also fail to respond to the students' communicative attempts, requiring them practice persistency or modifying their message

Activity Steps and Sample Language

This activity begins by showing students what they are going to make. It will be important to get students excited about making their own "slime." After showing students what you are going to be making you can ask them to make suggestions of what materials you might need. After all the materials have been gathered have students mix Borax and water together (sample language: "Get bowl," "Pour in," "Ready, set, go," "Stop," "No more pour," "Get more water," "Mix it," "Mix fast/slow"). Next, empty the Glitter Glue into a tub, add water, and mix (sample language: "Open glue," "Get glue," "Get water," "You mix it. Lastly, "Want help pour?", "I do it," "More glue," "Stop water," "Pour in," "Put in tub"). Have child mix in googly eyes and make shapes with the cookie cutters (sample language, "Put on eyes," "Make shape," "squishy shape," "Make more," "You do it," "Help me," "Look at shape," "I see glitter," "All done," "Little or big shape?").

APPENDIX F

Contents of the PluralPlus Companion Website

Fringe Vocabulary Worksheet

AAC Programming to Facilitate Communication Skills: Knowledge Skills Checklist

Technical Programming Training Checklist

Communication Demands and Opportunities Inventory

Communication Sample Form

Communication Sample Scoring Form

AAC Competency Skills Progress Report

Daily Data Collection Form by Activity

Daily Data Collection Form by Communicative Competency Goals

Sample Letter: "School-to-Home" Books

Index

Note: Page numbers in **bold** reference non-text material.